THE
GASTRITIS
HEALING
COOKBOOK

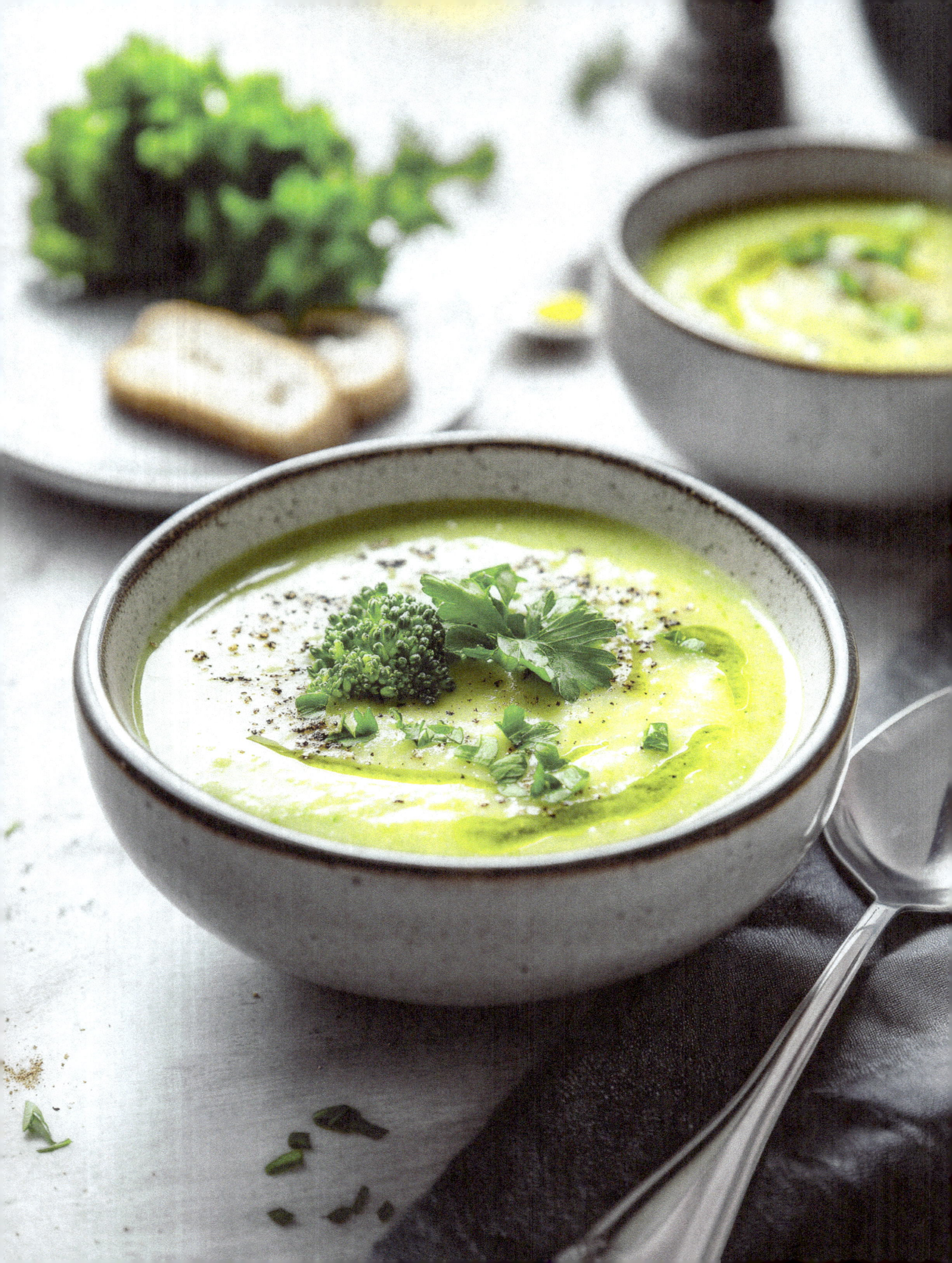

THE GASTRITIS HEALING COOKBOOK

125+ Delicious, Gastritis-Friendly Recipes to Soothe and Heal Your Stomach

L.G. CAPELLAN

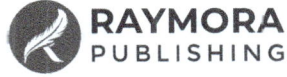

RAYMORA
PUBLISHING

Published by Raymora Publishing LLC.

Revised edition: May 2025

ISBN: 979-8-9926923-2-7

To the resilient spirit of every individual battling gastritis— may this book bring you comfort and healing.

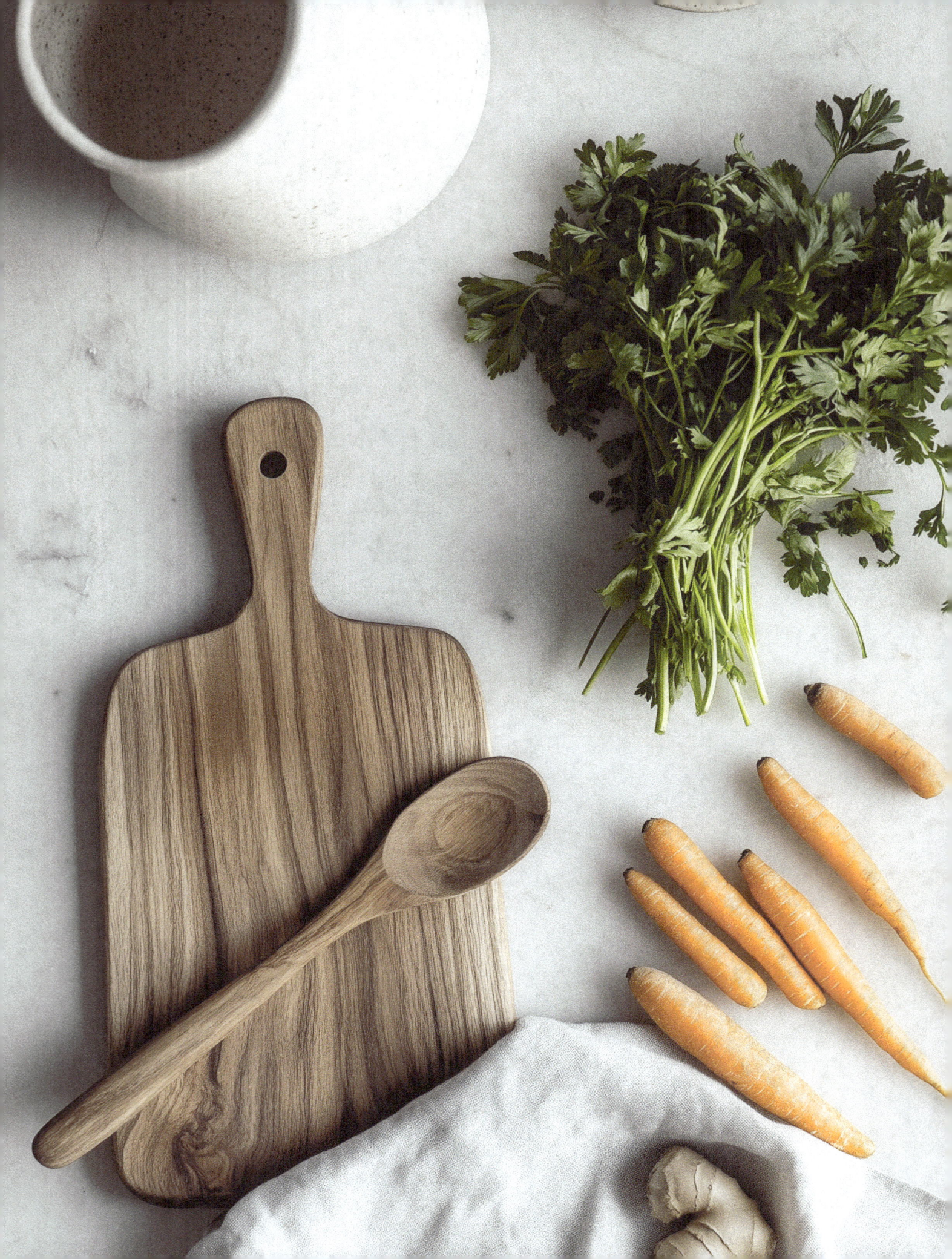

CONTENTS

INTRODUCTION

When I was first diagnosed with gastritis, I remember feeling overwhelmed as I looked through endless lists of foods to avoid. It seemed like all my favorite dishes were suddenly forbidden, and the joy of eating turned into a fear of dining. My kitchen, which had always been a place of comfort and creativity, now felt like a minefield where every ingredient threatened to cause pain.

I could still vividly remember the smells of garlic sautéing, the sizzle of onions in hot oil, and the comforting scent of cinnamon wafting from the oven—these were the aromas that once made my kitchen come alive. Standing in that same kitchen, now surrounded by the memories of those delicious meals, I felt a profound sense of loss. The ingredients that had inspired my cooking were now gathering dust on my shelves.

Each mealtime turned into a constant reminder of the foods I had to avoid. There was an almost palpable silence as I prepared yet another bland meal, missing the lively sounds of frying. All I heard was the soft sound of a knife cutting through boiled vegetables and tasteless chicken breast. My dining table, which used to be full of family chatter and laughter, now saw quiet, lonely dinners where the only sound was my fork and knife against the plate.

As the weeks turned into months, the dietary restrictions began to affect more than just my physical health; they started to wear down my emotional well-being and my social life. I found myself turning down invitations to eat out with a polite, yet heavy, heart. Eventually, my friends stopped asking, and I felt myself slipping into isolation, retreating further into a world shaped by my gastritis.

One particularly bleak evening, as I sat at my kitchen table facing yet another bland, uninspiring meal, I reached my breaking point. The mushy vegetables and watery soups stared back at me, a challenge I was no longer willing to accept without a fight. In that moment of despair, a rebellious thought ignited within me. Why should gastritis condemn me to a life without flavor? Was there really no balance between health and enjoyment?

Fueled by desperation and a profound craving for the flavors I missed, I decided to venture back into the world of cooking, but with a new approach. I pored over every piece of nutritional advice for gastritis I could find, determined to understand not just what I couldn't eat, but why. Armed with this knowledge, I began to experiment. If garlic was off the table, could a pinch of asafoetida provide that sharp kick? If lemon was too acidic, might lemon zest add a subtle tang to my dishes? I experimented tirelessly, mixing, seasoning, and tasting, transforming each 'safe' ingredient into a part of a richer culinary experience.

Little by little, I turned my kitchen from a place of restrictions into a space for culinary adventures. Every recipe I mastered felt like a victory, and every meal became a celebration of joy I had reclaimed. This cookbook is the culmination of that journey. It is more than just a collection of recipes; it's a manifesto for taking back your kitchen, one gastritis-friendly dish at a time.

Why This Cookbook?

After the release of my previous work, *The Gastritis Healing Book*, which laid down the foundational knowledge for managing gastritis, I realized the necessity for a more hands-on resource tailored to the kitchen. This cookbook fulfills that need—a practical companion designed to bring the principles from the previous book into your kitchen, transforming them into delicious, healing meals. It serves as a bridge from understanding gastritis to actively living well with it, providing recipes that complement the dietary advice and insights from the earlier work.

As I combined medical insights with culinary creativity, my goal was clear: to empower you to take control of your gastritis with every meal you prepare. This cookbook is about turning dietary restrictions into opportunities for gastronomic exploration, ensuring that you never feel deprived, even while following a strict diet. By offering recipes that minimize stomach irritation, it also enables you to experiment safely with new flavors and dishes, expanding your dietary options and enhancing your enjoyment of food.

Moreover, this cookbook is about more than just managing symptoms—it's about enriching your life. It's crafted to help you reconnect with the joy of cooking and eating, transforming mealtime into an opportunity for celebration and connection. Each recipe invites you to rediscover the pleasure of culinary creation, transforming potential limitations into a source of continual culinary delight.

By building on the foundation laid by my previous book, this cookbook aims to provide you with the tools to not only manage your condition but also to thrive despite it. Whether you're navigating food sensitivities, seeking variety, or just wanting to enjoy delicious, safe meals, this cookbook guides you through each step, ensuring a richer, more flavorful approach to a gastritis-friendly diet.

About the Recipes

IN THIS BOOK, YOU WILL FIND OVER 125 GASTRITIS-FRIENDLY RECIPES FOR EVERY MEAL OF THE DAY.

These recipes are specially designed to cater to different stages of managing gastritis, ensuring that you have suitable options whether you are seeking gentle, healing foods or aiming to maintain your digestive health during the more stable phases.

Each dish has been meticulously crafted to be both gluten-free and dairy-free, accommodating common dietary sensitivities and significantly broadening their suitability for various dietary needs.

To assist you in easily navigating through the cookbook and accurately identifying recipes according to the phase of your diet, we have introduced intuitive visual cues:

- **HEALING PHASE RECIPES** These are marked with a green line ——— below their names. Recipes in this category are formulated to be gentle on the stomach, aiding in the healing process by minimizing inflammation. They are ideal for those who are experiencing active symptoms or who are in the early stages of their treatment plan.

- **MAINTENANCE PHASE RECIPES** These feature a yellow line ——— below their names. These recipes are suitable for individuals who have moved past the acute phase of gastritis and are focused on maintaining their health. They are designed to continue supporting stomach health without the strict limitations required during the healing phase.

These visual markers ensure that you can quickly and effortlessly find the recipes that best meet your needs at any given time. From nutritious breakfasts to delectable dinners, each recipe is crafted to be safe and soothing while also adding variety and enjoyment to your diet.

PART ONE

GETTING STARTED

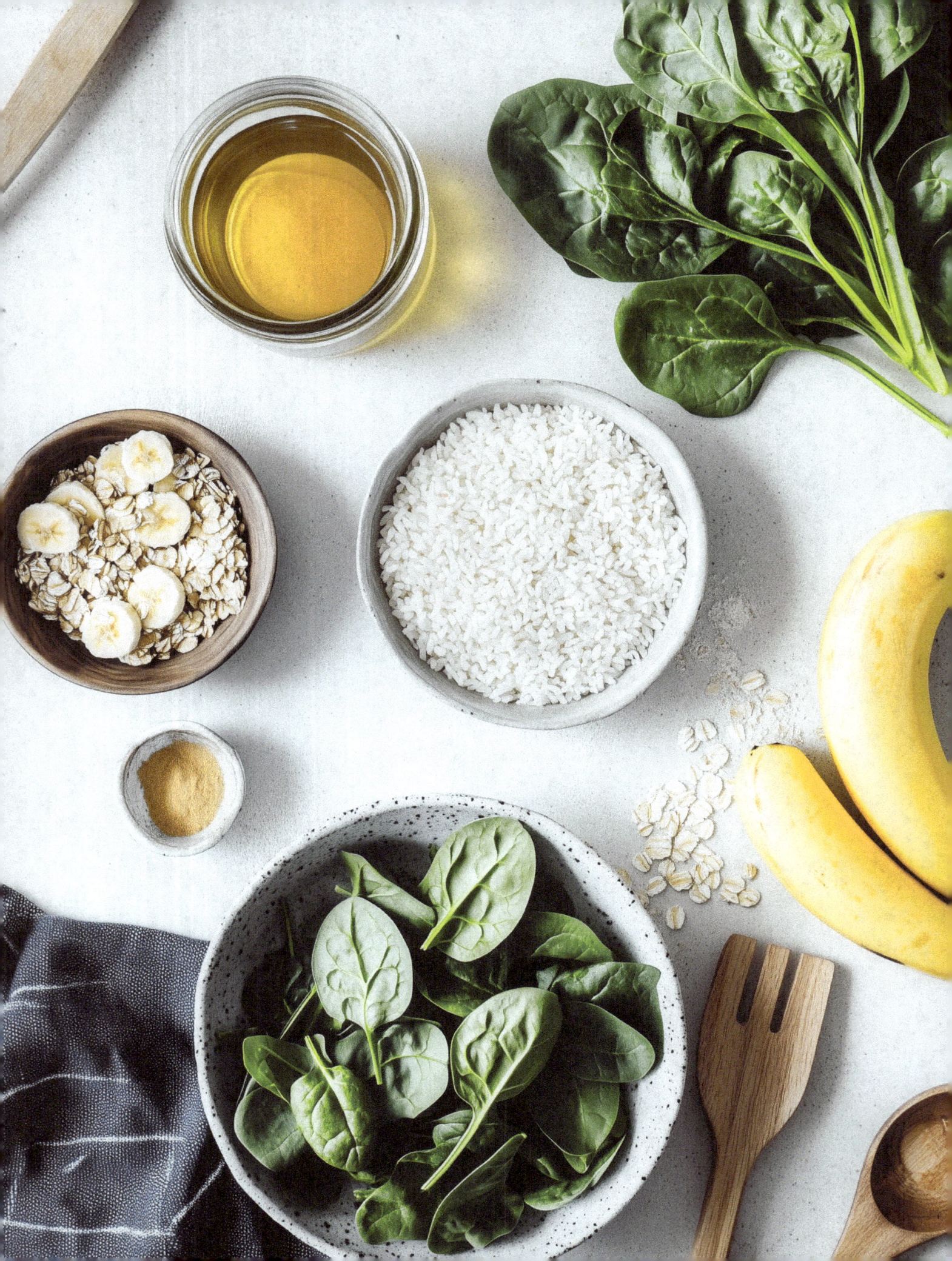

CHAPTER ONE

THE BASICS OF A GASTRITIS-FRIENDLY DIET

Navigating the world of food with gastritis can feel like walking through a minefield. Every meal, every bite, holds potential consequences that can either soothe or aggravate your stomach. This is why a deep understanding of gastritis and its dietary management is not just helpful—it's essential.

Gastritis, an inflammation of the stomach lining, can be triggered by various factors, including certain medications, *H. pylori* infection, alcohol, stress, and irregular eating habits. While addressing the root cause is crucial for managing the condition, following a gastritis-friendly diet is equally important for effective treatment.

The gastritis diet emphasizes avoiding foods known to trigger symptoms or cause stomach discomfort, such as spicy, acidic, fried, fatty, processed, and fast foods, along with alcohol, soft drinks, and caffeine. In contrast, a gastritis-friendly diet should prioritize low-acid, bland, and anti-inflammatory foods. Here's why:

- **LOW-ACID** The primary goal of adopting a low-acid diet is to minimize the activation of pepsinogen into pepsin—a digestive enzyme that can exacerbate stomach irritation when triggered by acidic foods such as tomatoes, citrus fruits, and vinegar-based dressings. In individuals with inflamed gastric tissues, this can lead to increased discomfort and prolonged healing times. By reducing the intake of acidic foods, a low-acid diet helps create a more conducive environment for healing by discouraging the activation of pepsin.

- **BLAND** A bland diet is essential for facilitating easier digestion, which is especially beneficial for individuals experiencing gastritis. This includes foods that are soft, not heavily seasoned, and low in fat, such as boiled potatoes, steamed vegetables, and lean meats like chicken or turkey breast. The primary purpose is to reduce the digestive system's workload, allowing the stomach to heal without the additional stress of breaking down complex or spicy foods that can cause irritation.

- **ANTI-INFLAMMATORY** The benefits of consuming anti-inflammatory foods are manifold. They not only help reduce the immediate inflammation typical of gastritis but also bolster the overall health and resilience of the digestive system. This is why incorporating antioxidant-rich fruits and vegetables into a gastritis-friendly diet is crucial—it soothes the gastrointestinal tract and supports the body's natural healing processes.

In the following sections, we will delve into these dietary principles in detail. You'll discover which foods aid in your healing process and learn why certain common foods can be harmful to those with gastritis. Armed with this knowledge, you'll be better equipped to manage your condition effectively, leading to a healthier digestive system and a more comfortable lifestyle.

The Different Phases of The Gastritis Diet

Managing gastritis through diet involves distinct phases, each tailored to address the specific needs of the healing process and long-term management of the condition. There are two main phases: the healing phase and the maintenance phase. Understanding these phases is crucial for effectively navigating your dietary choices, which will facilitate recovery and help maintain gastrointestinal health over the long term.

HEALING PHASE

The healing phase is critical for those newly diagnosed with gastritis or those experiencing severe symptoms. This initial stage is all about calming the stomach lining, reducing inflammation, and fostering an environment conducive to healing. It's a time for careful dietary management and lifestyle adjustments to give your body the support it needs to recover.

- **DIET FOCUS** Incorporate foods that are especially gentle on the stomach to support your healing during the critical initial phase of gastritis. This includes a selection of soft, easy-to-digest, and low-acid foods foods that won't aggravate the stomach lining.

- **AVOID** Strictly avoid irritants such as alcohol, caffeine, spicy foods, irritating vegetables, and acidic fruits (especially on an empty stomach). Additionally, it's advisable to avoid dairy products and fatty foods, as they can exacerbate symptoms.

- **OBJECTIVE** The goal during this phase is to minimize stomach irritation and inflammation to allow the stomach lining to recover more quickly. This may require a highly restrictive diet, depending on the severity of symptoms and individual reactions to different foods.

MAINTENANCE PHASE

After successfully controlling the initial symptoms of gastritis, the maintenance phase plays a crucial role in managing the condition over the long term and preventing its recurrence. This stage marks a transition from strict dietary control to a more balanced approach, where the goal is sustained stomach health.

- **DIET FOCUS** Gradually reintroduce a broader range of foods while monitoring the body's response. This phase still emphasizes foods that promote digestive health but allows more flexibility. You can slowly start to include more fibrous vegetables, fruits with a pH below 5, and possibly small amounts of foods that were off-limits during the healing phase.

- **OBJECTIVE** The aim is to maintain a diet that supports ongoing stomach health and prevents the aggravation of gastritis symptoms. This involves a personalized approach, adjusting dietary choices based on ongoing feedback from your body. It's about finding a balance that allows you to enjoy a varied diet while keeping your gastritis in check.

By strategically navigating these two phases, you can effectively manage your condition, reduce symptoms during flare-ups, and maintain your digestive health over the long term. Regular consultations with a healthcare provider or dietitian are recommended to tailor the diet appropriately and ensure that nutritional needs are met throughout each phase.

Trigger Foods to Eliminate and Avoid

When it comes to managing gastritis through diet, there is a broad spectrum of foods to avoid and eliminate from your diet. However, it's crucial to acknowledge that gastritis affects individuals differently, meaning what might trigger symptoms in one person could be tolerable for another. Therefore, it's essential to categorize foods into distinct groups: the definitive NO list and those recommended to avoid.

THE BIG NO LIST

This category includes foods that generally have a high potential to irritate the stomach and exacerbate the symptoms of gastritis, regardless of the individual. These food items directly or indirectly harm the stomach lining by increasing acid secretion or causing irritation. Here's a list of foods you consider to eliminate from your diet:

- **ALCOHOL** All types of alcoholic beverages, including beer, wine, and spirits, can irritate and inflame the stomach lining. Alcohol can weaken the protective mucous layer of the stomach, making the delicate tissues more vulnerable to acid. Beer and wine have the added effect of increasing stomach acid production, compounding the risk of irritation and leading to more severe gastritis symptoms.[1]

- **COFFEE AND OTHER CAFFEINATED BEVERAGES** Caffeine is a potent stimulant that can lead to an increase in stomach acid secretion. Regular consumption of coffee, tea, and other caffeinated drinks can contribute to gastric distress by heightening acid production, thereby aggravating the condition of those with gastritis.[2]

- **SPICY AND IRRITATING FOODS** Ingredients such as hot peppers, chili, black or red peppers, hot sauce, onions, and garlic are notorious for aggravating the lining of the stomach. These foods can cause a burning sensation and lead to inflammation in an already sensitive stomach. Condiments like ketchup, mayonnaise, and mustard also fall into this category because they often contain vinegar and spices that can trigger symptoms.

- **HIGHLY ACIDIC FOODS** Includes citrus fruits, tomatoes, and fermented foods like sauerkraut and vinegar-based pickles, all known for their high acidity. These foods can activate pepsin, an enzyme in the stomach that, when active, can contribute to the degradation of the stomach lining, exacerbating inflammation and pain. (Later, we'll discuss how to consume some acidic fruits safely.)

- **SODA AND SOFT DRINKS** The carbonation in sodas and other soft drinks introduces carbonic acid into the stomach. Additionally, these beverages often contain other acidulants like citric acid and phosphoric acid, which can further activate pepsin and irritate the gastric lining, leading to increased symptoms of gastritis.

- **VINEGAR** Vinegar, whether it's apple cider, balsamic, or red wine vinegar, is highly acidic. Its consumption can significantly increase the activity of pepsin, which in turn can aggravate the inflammation in the stomach lining, making gastritis symptoms worse.

- **CHOCOLATE** Chocolate contains a substance called methylxanthine, which relaxes the lower esophageal sphincter (LES). This relaxation can allow stomach acid to escape into the esophagus, causing acid reflux. Additionally, methylxanthine stimulates the stomach to produce more acid, a double threat for those with gastritis.[3]

Eliminating these foods from your diet can be a crucial step in managing gastritis and reducing flare-ups. While it may seem restrictive, it's necessary to avoid these kinds of foods to kick-start the healing process of your stomach. Additionally, with the right strategies and substitutions, you can still enjoy a varied and satisfying diet without the foods that trigger your symptoms.

THE RECOMMENDED TO AVOID LIST

This category includes foods that may not harm everyone with gastritis but are commonly known to cause gastrointestinal discomfort. Therefore, they are best limited or completely avoided during the initial phase of managing gastritis. These foods include:

- **DAIRY PRODUCTS** While some individuals might tolerate low-fat dairy options such as non-fat yogurt, skim milk, and certain low-fat cheeses the majority of dairy products contain beta-casein A1, a protein that recent studies suggest may aggravate gastrointestinal symptoms and contribute to intestinal inflammation.[4]

- **GLUTEN-CONTAINING FOODS** Gluten, a protein found in wheat, barley, and rye, can trigger inflammatory responses and contribute to digestive discomfort and exacerbation of gastrointestinal symptoms in some individuals. Common sources of gluten include bread, pasta, cereals, and baked goods.[5]

- **WHOLE GRAINS, BEANS, AND LEGUMES** While these foods are rich in fiber and essential nutrients, they can be challenging for those suffering from gastritis. Their high fiber content can lead to increased gas production, bloating, and stomach discomfort.

- **FRIED AND FATTY FOODS** Due to their high fat content, these foods tend to slow gastric emptying, which can increase the likelihood of acid reflux and stomach irritation. It's advisable to avoid foods like fried chicken, French fries, and other unhealthy, fatty foods.

- **PROCESSED FOODS** Often high in additives and low in nutritional value, processed foods can trigger inflammation and exacerbate digestive symptoms. Avoiding items such as canned soups, frozen dinners, and processed snacks can help reduce these negative effects.

Avoiding these commonly problematic foods during the initial phase of gastritis management can significantly aid in symptom relief and promote healing. As healing progresses, some of these foods may be reintroduced in moderation, but starting with a careful approach helps set the foundation for long-term digestive health

Gastritis-Friendly Foods to Include

Incorporating the right foods into your diet is crucial for managing gastritis and supporting the healing process. By focusing on options that are gentle on the stomach, you can help reduce inflammation and support your path to recovery. Here are some foods to include

- **LOW-ACID FRUITS** Include bananas, papaya, melons, watermelon, dragon fruit, Bosc and Asian pears, and Medjool and Deglet dates, which are less acidic and rich in antioxidants. Acidic fruits like berries, mangoes, peaches, and apples are generally not recommended, especially on an empty stomach. However, their acidity can be neutralized in smoothies made with plant-based milks such as almond or coconut milk.

- **COOKED VEGETABLES** Most vegetables are suitable, with the exception of tomatoes, garlic, and onions. Always cook vegetables to make them easier on the stomach, and avoid raw vegetables initially, as they can be rough on the stomach lining and more difficult to digest.

- **LEAN PROTEINS** Skinless chicken or turkey breasts, white fish, egg whites, and tofu are excellent sources of essential nutrients and amino acids while being low in fat, which helps prevent aggravation of gastritis symptoms. Depending on your tolerance, you might also be able to include small amounts of slightly fatty options, such as salmon or egg yolks, as long as they are prepared in a gentle manner.

- **GENTLE GRAINS** Quick-cooking or instant oatmeal and white rice are preferable among grains as they contain less fiber, making them easier to digest. These options are less likely to irritate the stomach and can provide a soothing, easily digestible source of carbohydrates.

- **ROOT VEGETABLES** Potatoes, sweet potatoes, yams, cassava (yuca), and malanga (taro) are energy-rich and generally less likely to cause stomach irritation when cooked without added fats. These root vegetables are easy on the stomach and can be a soothing addition to your diet, providing essential nutrients without exacerbating gastritis symptoms.

- **HEALTHY FATS** Olive oil, coconut oil, and avocado oil are excellent sources of healthy fats. They are also ideal for cooking, particularly coconut and avocado oil, which are stable at high temperatures. However, due to their fat content, they should be used sparingly and in small quantities.

- **CONDIMENTS** Gastritis-friendly seasonings such as oregano, rosemary, thyme, parsley, cilantro, basil, ginger, turmeric, cumin, and liquid aminos or coconut aminos can enhance flavor without irritating the stomach. These options provide a way to add taste to your meals while keeping your stomach comfortable.

- **NATURAL SWEETENERS** Opt for pure maple syrup, monk fruit, and stevia as healthier alternatives to refined sugar. These sweeteners provide a touch of sweetness without negatively affecting your digestive system, helping to maintain a gastritis-friendly diet. Honey can also be used, but it should be properly neutralized due to its naturally low pH around 4.

Incorporating these gastritis-friendly foods into your diet can help manage symptoms and promote healing of the stomach lining. It is important to observe how your body reacts to different foods and adjust your diet accordingly. With careful planning and consideration, you can enjoy a varied and nutritious diet that supports your digestive health.

Tips for Preparing and Cooking Your Food

The gastritis diet is not only about what to eat but also how to prepare it. Proper food preparation and cooking methods are vital to avoid exacerbating the condition. Follow these key tips to prepare meals that promote digestion and alleviate stomach discomfort.

- **PEEL AND DE-SEED FRUITS AND VEGETABLES** Removing the skins and seeds from fruits and certain vegetables can aid digestion, particularly beneficial during acute gastritis episodes. Skins are often high in fiber, which can be tough on a irritated stomach. Additionally, peeling can remove residues of pesticides or waxes, enhancing safety and digestibility.

- **BLENDING AND PUREEING** Transforming hard or fibrous vegetables and fruits into smoothies or soups can make nutrients more accessible and lessen stomach irritation. Opt for easily digestible choices like mashed potatoes, sweet potatoes, cassava, or pureed carrots, and use plant-based milks to create smooth blends that support stomach health without triggering symptoms.

- **MARINATING** Tenderize meats by marinating in mild, non-acidic solutions. Avoid acidic components like vinegar or citrus, which can worsen gastritis. Instead, opt for broths or mild oils like olive oil to soften the meat fibers without adding acidity.

- **GENTLE COOKING METHODS** Employ cooking techniques that are kind to the stomach lining, such as steaming, boiling, poaching, slow cooking, and sautéing with minimal oil. These methods help preserve the nutritional integrity of foods while minimizing the risk of irritation. While baking, grilling, and air frying are generally suitable, ensure that food remains soft and not overly crispy to avoid irritating the stomach lining. Avoid high-heat methods like deep-frying or high-temperature grilling that can produce harmful compounds and make foods overly hard.

- **CONTROL COOKING TIME** Balancing cooking time is crucial to ensure that foods are soft enough to be easily digestible yet retain their nutritional value. Properly cooked foods support digestive health and contribute to the healing of the stomach lining. Adjust cooking times based on the type of food and preparation method to optimize both digestibility and nutrient absorption.

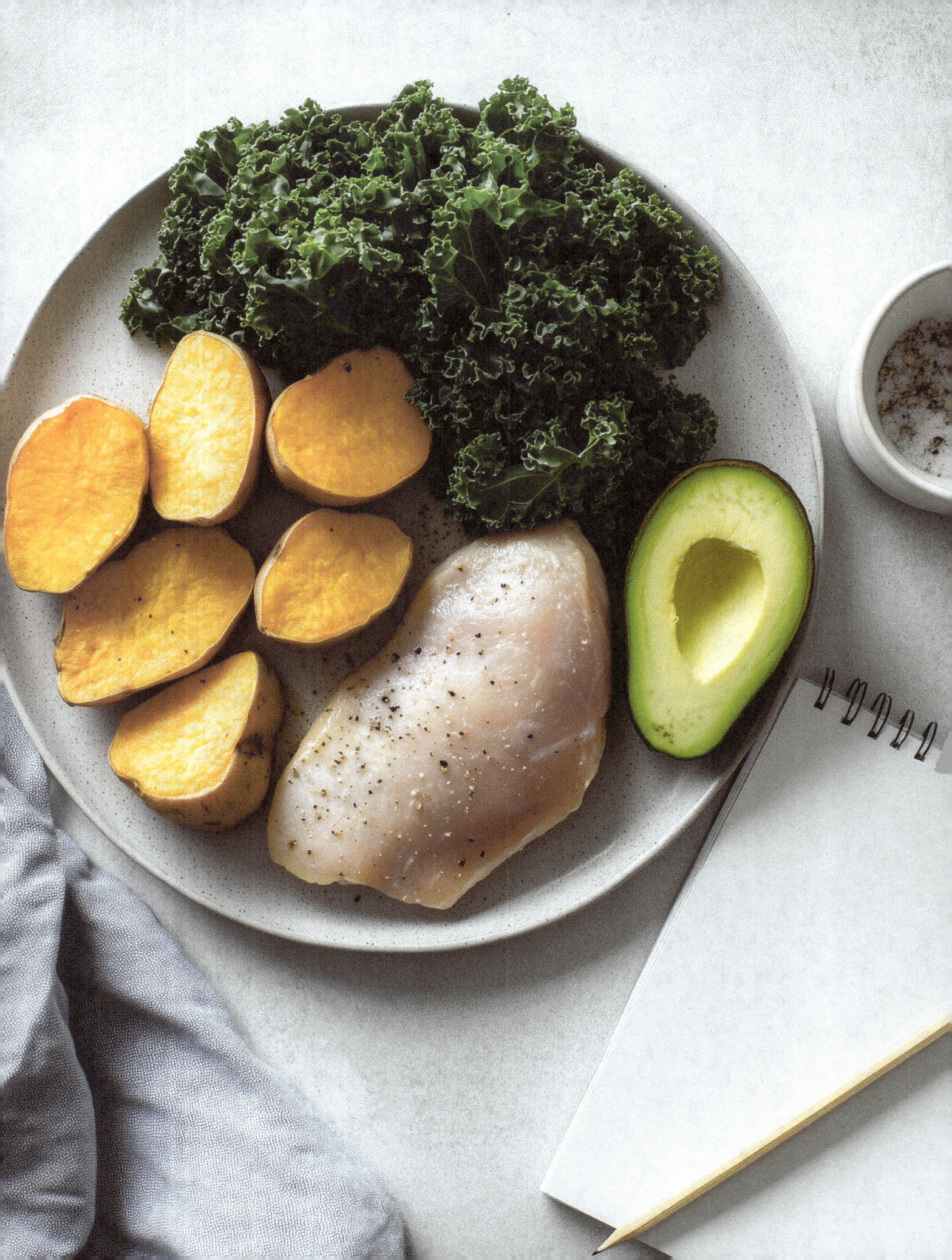

CHAPTER TWO

MENU PLANNING AND MEAL PREP STRATEGIES

Embarking on a journey to manage gastritis through diet is not just about avoiding certain foods—it's about embracing a lifestyle that supports your digestive health at every meal. Personalized meal planning is a cornerstone of this approach, tailored to meet your individual dietary needs and preferences. By customizing your diet, you can effectively mitigate symptoms, promote healing, and maintain long-term gastrointestinal health.

In this chapter, we delve into the practical aspects of creating your own meal plan using the recipes provided in this book. These recipes are not only gastritis-friendly but are also designed to be versatile and adaptable, making it easier for you to prepare delicious and soothing meals every day. By integrating these recipes into your meal planning, you streamline the process, ensuring that managing your diet becomes both enjoyable and sustainable.

As we move forward, you'll learn how to harness the power of these recipes to construct a meal plan that not only meets your nutritional needs but also fits seamlessly into your daily routine. From understanding the basic principles of meal planning to implementing advanced meal prep strategies, this chapter will provide you with all the tools you need to take control of your gastritis through thoughtful and effective dietary management.

Creating a Personalized Meal Plan

Embarking on the creation of a personalized meal plan empowers you to take control of your gastritis management through diet. This process involves identifying which foods soothe and which aggravate your condition, allowing you to assemble meals that are not only nourishing but also comforting.

ASSESSING DIETARY NEEDS

The first step in personalizing your meal plan involves an acute observation of how your body responds to different foods. Start by maintaining a detailed food diary to document your daily intake and note any gastritis symptoms that follow. This record will help you identify patterns and pinpoint specific foods that trigger your symptoms, providing a clear direction for adjustments in your diet.

It's also important to note that effective management of gastritis goes beyond avoiding triggers; it includes optimizing your nutritional intake to support the healing process and reduce inflammation. Consult with a healthcare provider or a dietitian to gain a comprehensive understanding of your nutritional needs. This includes determining the right balance of macronutrients—proteins, fats, and carbohydrates—and ensuring adequate intake of essential vitamins and minerals that foster recovery and health.

SETTING UP YOUR MEAL PLAN TEMPLATE

A well-structured meal plan template is crucial for organizing your meals. This template should include sections for each day of the week, with slots for breakfast, lunch, dinner, and snacks. Here's a simple breakdown of what your template might look like:

MONDAY
Breakfast
Mid-morning Snack
Lunch
Afternoon Snack
Dinner

Continue this format through the week, ensuring you have ample space to note down specific meals and their ingredients. This organizational tool will not only help you visualize your weekly food intake but also assist in grocery shopping and prep scheduling.

RECIPE SELECTION

Once your meal plan template is ready, the crucial next step is selecting the right recipes to fill it. This task isn't just about picking meals that you enjoy; it's about choosing wisely based on your unique dietary needs and how certain foods impact your gastritis. Here's how to ensure that your recipe selection is both strategic and supportive of your health goals:

1. **ANALYZE DIETARY TRIGGERS** Start by reviewing the dietary triggers and sensitivities you've identified in your initial assessment. Each recipe choice should be scrutinized through this lens—ensuring it does not contain ingredients known to aggravate your symptoms. For instance, if broccoli or bananas trigger your gastritis, you'll want to avoid recipes that use these as primary ingredients.

2. **EVALUATE NUTRITIONAL CONTENT** Focus on recipes that not only avoid triggers but also contribute to your overall nutritional needs. Recipes should be balanced with adequate proteins, healthy fats, and carbohydrates to support your body's healing and energy needs.

3. **COMPILE A DIVERSE SET** To prevent dietary monotony and ensure a broad range of nutrients, compile a diverse set of recipes. Include various cuisines and cooking styles that fit within your dietary guidelines, expanding your palate and keeping mealtime interesting and enjoyable.

By thoughtfully selecting recipes based on these criteria, you can fill your meal plan with meals that not only satisfy your taste buds but also nourish and heal your body. This strategic approach ensures that every meal contributes positively towards managing your gastritis, paving the way for more comfortable and enjoyable dining experiences.

INCORPORATION INTO MEAL PLANS

With your curated list of recipes ready, the next step is to strategically integrate these into your meal plan. This process is essential for ensuring your diet meets your nutritional needs, fits your lifestyle, and addresses the challenges of managing gastritis effectively.

- **BALANCE YOUR NUTRIENTS** Distribute recipes throughout the week to ensure each day includes a balanced mix of macronutrients—proteins, carbohydrates, and fats—along with essential vitamins and minerals. This balance supports optimal energy levels and overall health, crucial for managing gastritis symptoms.

- **CONSIDER MEAL TIMING** Align meal times with your body's natural rhythms and daily schedule. Eating regularly helps regulate stomach acid levels and prevent discomfort associated with irregular eating habits.

- **DIVERSIFY YOUR MEALS** Ensure variety in your meals to prevent monotony and provide a broad spectrum of nutrients. Incorporating different textures, flavors, and ingredients makes meals more enjoyable and can positively influence digestion and health.

- **PREP IN ADVANCE** Prepare ingredients or entire meals ahead of time to improve efficiency and adherence to your diet. This might include chopping vegetables, marinating proteins, or preparing dishes like stews and casseroles that store well.

- **MAINTAIN FLEXIBILITY** Allow flexibility in your meal plan for adjustments based on dietary responses or changes in your routine. This adaptability ensures your meal plan remains practical and responsive to your daily needs.

By integrating these strategies into your meal plan, you create a diet that is not only nutritionally balanced but also tailored to manage gastritis effectively. This approach helps in symptom management and enhances your dietary experience, making it sustainable and beneficial long-term.

ADAPTATION FOR TOLERANCE AND TASTE

The final step in creating your personalized meal plan is to adapt the selected recipes to fit your unique dietary tolerances and taste preferences. This customization is key to ensuring that your meal plan not only supports your health but is also enjoyable and sustainable over the long term.

1. **IDENTIFYING SUBSTITUTIONS** Begin by identifying any ingredients in your chosen recipes that you need to avoid due to intolerance, allergies, or personal dislike. For each of these, find suitable substitutes that do not compromise the flavor or nutritional value of the dish. For example, if you are sensitive to leeks, consider using asafoetida, or aromatic herbs like basil or oregano.

2. **ADJUSTING FLAVORS** Tailor the recipes to suit your flavor preferences. If you prefer milder dishes, reduce the use of spices or opt for herbs that contribute flavor without adding heat. Conversely, if you enjoy more flavorful dishes but need to avoid certain irritants, experiment with gastritis-friendly spices and herbs that can enhance taste without causing discomfort.

3. **MODIFYING COOKING METHODS** Some recipes may require adjustments in cooking methods to make them more suitable for your condition. For instance, if a recipe calls for grilling, you might adapt it to baking or steaming to make it lighter and easier on your stomach.

4. **PORTION SIZES** Adjust portion sizes according to your digestive comfort. Most people with gastritis find it easier to manage smaller, more frequent meals rather than larger ones, which can overwhelm the digestive system and exacerbate symptoms.

5. **MEAL COMBINATIONS** Consider the interactions between different components of each meal. Certain food combinations, such as a large amount of carbohydrates paired with a protein-rich meal, might be harder to digest or too heavy. Customize your meal plan to include combinations that are harmonious and promote easier digestion. This careful pairing can help manage gastritis symptoms more effectively by reducing digestive stress.

6. **EXPERIMENTATION AND FEEDBACK** The process of adapting recipes is often iterative. As you try different substitutions and modifications, pay close attention to how you feel afterwards. Use this feedback to make further adjustments, gradually refining each recipe to perfectly match your dietary needs and preferences.

By taking the time to adapt recipes for tolerance and taste, you create a meal plan that is not only effective in managing your gastritis but also pleasurable to follow. This personalized approach encourages adherence to the dietary changes, making it easier to maintain these healthy habits over time.

Meal Prep Tips and Recommendations

Efficient meal preparation is key to successfully managing gastritis through diet. This section provides practical tips and recommendations to streamline your cooking process, ensuring that your gastritis-friendly meals are not only easy to prepare but also suitable for your lifestyle. We'll cover batch cooking, effective storage solutions, and time-saving kitchen gadgets.

BATCH COOKING AND STORAGE

This method involves preparing large quantities of food at once, which can be stored and used throughout the week. It is particularly beneficial for those with busy schedules or for anyone needing consistent access to suitable meals. Proper storage is also crucial to maintain the freshness and nutritional value of your cooked meals. Here's how to manage this effectively:

- **PLAN YOUR SESSIONS** Identify recipes from the book suitable for batch cooking—such as soups or rice dishes—and set aside a few hours for cooking.

- **EFFICIENT USE OF INGREDIENTS** Optimize your ingredient usage by preparing multiple dishes that share similar ingredients, reducing waste and saving money.

- **COOKING PROCESS** Use large pots, slow cookers, or pressure cookers to handle larger quantities more efficiently and ensure even cooking.

- **COOLING DOWN** Allow food to cool completely before storing to prevent bacterial growth and maintain food safety.

- **PORTIONING** Divide meals into portion-sized containers. This not only makes it easier to manage meal sizes but also simplifies reheating.

- **LABELING** Label your containers with the contents and the date they were cooked to aid in stock rotation and ensure older meals are used first.

- **FREEZING** Most batch-cooked meals are suitable for freezing. Store them in airtight containers or freezer bags to prevent freezer burn and extend their shelf life.

- **REFRIGERATION** Adjust your refrigerator's temperature settings to ensure optimal freshness. Keep cooked and raw ingredients separate to avoid cross-contamination.

- **DRY STORAGE** Invest in good quality airtight containers for dry ingredients like grains, herb, and spices. Store them in a cool, dry place to extend their shelf life and maintain flavor.

- **USE OF SPACE** Utilize organizational tools such as shelf organizers, lazy Susans, and clear storage containers to make it easy to see and access what you need quickly.

TIME-SAVING KITCHEN GADGETS

Incorporate gadgets that can save time and simplify the cooking process:

- **FOOD PROCESSORS** Quickly chop, slice, or grate vegetables, which is especially helpful for preparing large batches of food.

- **SLOW COOKERS AND PRESSURE COOKERS** These are ideal for making stews, soups, and tender cooked meats with minimal active cooking time, allowing you to set them up and then focus on other tasks.

- **RICE COOKERS** Perfect for cooking grains without needing to monitor the stove, providing consistent results every time.

- **BLENDERS** Essential for making smoothies or pureeing soups, which are easy on the stomach for those with gastritis.

By utilizing these meal prep tips, storage solutions, and time-saving gadgets, you can make managing your gastritis through diet more practical and less time-consuming, allowing you to focus more on enjoying your meals and less on the preparation.

Setting Up Your Kitchen

A well-organized kitchen equipped with the right tools and ingredients is key to making meal preparation for gastritis management efficient and stress-free. This section offers guidance on setting up your kitchen to support your dietary needs effectively, focusing on the essential tools, pantry staples, and organization strategies.

ESSENTIAL TOOLS

Having the right tools at your disposal can greatly simplify the preparation of gastritis-friendly meals. Here are some essential kitchen tools that can help:

- **KNIVES** A good set of sharp knives is crucial for efficient food prep. Include a chef's knife, a paring knife, and a serrated knife to handle different types of cutting tasks.

- **CUTTING BOARDS** Have multiple cutting boards to prevent cross-contamination between raw and cooked foods.

- **MIXING BOWLS** A set of mixing bowls in various sizes is useful for preparing ingredients and mixing them.

- **MEASURING CUPS AND SPOONS** Accurate measuring tools ensure that recipes are followed precisely, which is particularly important for maintaining the balance of ingredients in gastritis-friendly recipes.

- **POTS AND PANS** Invest in a non-stick skillet, a large pot for soups and stews, and a medium saucepan. Consider materials like stainless steel or ceramic, which are durable and easy to clean.

PANTRY STAPLES

Keeping your pantry stocked with certain staples can help you whip up meals quickly without the constant need for fresh groceries. Here are some pantry essentials for those managing gastritis:

- **GRAINS** White rice and quick-cooking oats are versatile and easy on the stomach.

- **HERBS AND SPICES** Maintain a variety of gastritis-friendly options such as oregano, thyme, rosemary, basil, ginger, and turmeric to add flavor without causing irritation.

- **BROTHS AND STOCKS** Opt for low-sodium vegetable or chicken broths that exclude irritating ingredients like onion and garlic. These can form the foundation for many soothing soups and dishes, providing flavor without aggravation.

- **HEALTHY OILS** Such as olive oil or avocado oil, which are great for cooking and dressings.

- **NON-DAIRY MILKS** Almond, coconut, or oat milk can be used in cooking and baking or enjoyed on their own.

ORGANIZING YOUR SPACE

An organized kitchen can streamline your cooking process, making it quicker and more enjoyable. Here's how to effectively organize your space:

- **ZONE ORGANIZATION** Divide your kitchen into functional zones. Keep all your baking items together, and place cooking spices near the stove or in an easily accessible spot.

- **USE CLEAR CONTAINERS** Store ingredients in clear, airtight containers to keep them fresh and make it easy to see what you have at a glance.

- **MAXIMIZE VERTICAL SPACE** Use shelf risers and hanging racks to maximize vertical storage space in cabinets.

- **FREQUENT USE ITEMS** Keep frequently used items within easy reach. This might mean having oils, salts, and frequently used spices on a shelf above your cooking area.

- **LABEL EVERYTHING** Label shelves and containers to make it easier to find what you need without having to search through every cabinet.

By setting up your kitchen with the right tools, staples, and organizational systems, you can make the process of preparing gastritis-friendly meals as efficient and stress-free as possible, allowing you more time to enjoy your meals and less time worrying about preparation.

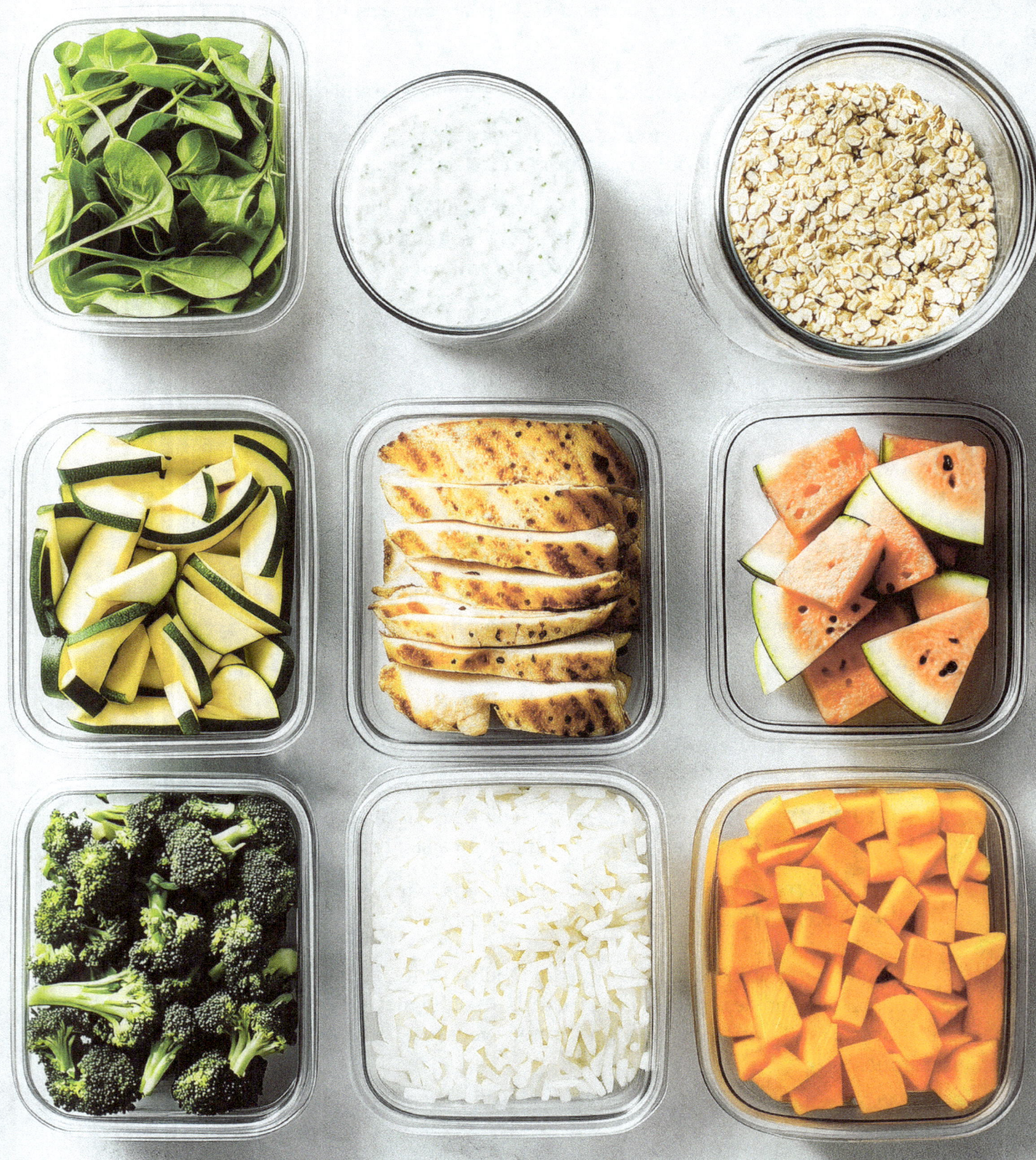

CHAPTER THREE

THE HEALING AND MAINTENANCE PHASE MEAL PLANS

I f you've ever felt overwhelmed by the process of crafting a meal plan—especially one focused on managing a specific health issue like gastritis—you're not alone. As someone who has navigated the choppy waters of gastritis myself, I understand the challenges of creating a health-focused meal plan from scratch. But worry not—I've designed this chapter to be your compass, guiding you through the healing and maintenance phases of gastritis with meal plans that are both nourishing and healing.

It's important to note that the meal plans provided here for the healing and maintenance phases are not one-size-fits-all. Feel free to use them as starting points to inspire and create plans tailored to the specific stages of your gastritis diet, adjusting them to better suit your unique health needs and tolerances.

As you move from the healing to the maintenance phase meal plan, remember that each step should be guided by your symptoms and tolerance. Monitoring how your body responds as you introduce new foods and adjust your diet is crucial. This careful approach will help you identify potential triggers and tailor your diet to ensure the best outcomes for your health.

Meal Plan for the Healing Phase

	DAY 1
Breakfast	Pumpkin Pancakes (p. 44)
Mid-morning Snack	Banana Avocado Smoothie (p. 62)
Lunch	Turkey Stroganoff with Roasted Broccoli (p. 76, 114)
Afternoon Snack	Baked Zucchini Fries (p. 124)
Dinner	Salmon Patties with Cauliflower Purée (p. 74, 120)

DAY 2	
Breakfast	French Toast (p. 54)
Mid-morning Snack	Pear Ginger Smoothie (p. 153)
Lunch	Sweet Potato Chicken Nuggets (p. 70)
Afternoon Snack	Crispy Carrot Chips (p. 134)
Dinner	Butternut Squash Soup (p. 92)

DAY 3	
Breakfast	Sweet Potato Pancakes (p. 50)
Mid-morning Snack	Melon Smoothie (p. 149)
Lunch	Creamy Broccoli Potato Soup (p. 89)
Afternoon Snack	Pumpkin Donuts (p. 137)
Dinner	Almond Crusted Chicken (p. 73)

DAY 4	
Breakfast	Crustless Spinach Quiche (p. 60)
Mid-morning Snack	Jasmine Milk Tea (p. 157)
Lunch	Chicken Ramen Bowl (p. 97)
Afternoon Snack	Broccoli Tots (p. 125)
Dinner	Herb Shrimp Pasta (p. 71)

DAY 5	
Breakfast	Zucchini Breakfast Bread (p. 61)
Mid-morning Snack	Chicory Latte (p. 154)
Lunch	Korean Rice Bowl (p. 100)
Afternoon Snack	Baked Yuca Fries (p. 141)
Dinner	Stuffed Cabbage Rolls (p. 91)

DAY 6	
Breakfast	Overnight Oats (p. 45)
Mid-morning Snack	Papaya Aloe Vera Smoothie (p. 156)
Lunch	Grilled Shrimp Skewers with Cauliflower Purée (p. 103, 120)
Afternoon Snack	Sweet Potato Brownies (p. 139)
Dinner	Creamy Macaroni Pasta (p. 94)

DAY 7	
Breakfast	Pumpkin Waffles (p. 47)
Mid-morning Snack	Banana Mango Smoothie (p. 146)
Lunch	Creamy Chicken Kale Soup (p. 101)
Afternoon Snack	Gingerbread Cookies (p. 135)
Dinner	Butternut Squash Pasta (p. 104)

SHOPPING LIST FOR THE HEALING PHASE MEAL PLAN

POULTRY AND EGGS

- ☐ 4 boneless, skinless chicken breasts (about 1½ pounds or 680 g)
- ☐ 2 ½ pounds (about 1,134 g) lean ground turkey breast
- ☐ 1 pound (about 450 g) ground chicken breast
- ☐ 23 large eggs

SEAFOOD

- ☐ 1 can (14.75 oz or 420 g) salmon
- ☐ 2 pounds (about 900 g) large shrimp

PRODUCE

- ☐ 1 large pumpkin (for purée) or 2 (15 oz or 425 g) cans pumpkin purée
- ☐ 2 large sweet potatoes
- ☐ 2 medium butternut squash (about 2½ pounds or 1,134 g)
- ☐ 12 medium carrots
- ☐ 4 celery stalks
- ☐ 2 large leeks
- ☐ 2 medium heads broccoli (about 1⅔ pounds or 750 g)
- ☐ 5 medium potatoes
- ☐ 2 medium heads cauliflower (about 1⅓ pounds or 600 g)
- ☐ 5 medium zucchinis
- ☐ 1 pound (about 450 g) mushrooms (button or baby bella)
- ☐ 1 large bunch spinach (about 7 cups)
- ☐ 1 small bunch kale
- ☐ 1 small bunch parsley
- ☐ 1 small bunch fresh basil

- ☐ 1 small golden beet
- ☐ 1 small head cabbage
- ☐ 2 lemons (for zest)
- ☐ 1 lime (optional, for zest)
- ☐ 1 small bunch fresh cilantro
- ☐ 1 small bunch fresh thyme
- ☐ 1 piece fresh ginger root
- ☐ 2 ripe avocados
- ☐ 2 medium bananas
- ☐ 1 small cantaloupe
- ☐ 2 ripe Bosc pears
- ☐ 1 small papaya
- ☐ 1 large mango
- ☐ ¼ pound (about 1 cup) blueberries, strawberries, or mixed berries

NUTS, SEEDS, AND GRAINS

- ☐ 1 (22 oz or 620 g) package gluten-free all-purpose flour
- ☐ 1 package gluten-free angel hair pasta
- ☐ 1 package gluten-free macaroni pasta
- ☐ 1 package gluten-free pasta (penne, rotini, or fusilli)
- ☐ 1 small package gluten-free breadcrumbs
- ☐ 1 small package quick-cooking or instant oats
- ☐ 1 package rice noodles
- ☐ 1 medium package white rice
- ☐ 1 gluten-free loaf
- ☐ 1 small package tapioca pearls (boba)
- ☐ 1 (16 oz or 450 g) package almond flour
- ☐ 1 (8 oz or 225 g) package coconut flour
- ☐ 1 small jar nut butter of choice
- ☐ 1 (8 oz or 225 g) package walnuts
- ☐ 1 small package nutritional yeast

OTHERS

- ☐ 1 gallon (128 oz or 3.78 L) unsweetened almond milk
- ☐ 1 liter (34 oz or 1 L) unsweetened coconut milk
- ☐ 1 can (13.5 oz or 400 mL) lite coconut milk

PANTRY ITEMS

- ☐ Maple syrup or honey
- ☐ Arrowroot flour or potato starch
- ☐ Baking powder
- ☐ Baking soda
- ☐ Liquid aminos or coconut aminos
- ☐ Unflavored gelatin
- ☐ Chicory root powder
- ☐ Carob powder
- ☐ Xanthan gum (if not included in the gluten-free flour)
- ☐ Olive oil
- ☐ Coconut oil
- ☐ Sesame oil
- ☐ Avocado oil (or odorless coconut oil)
- ☐ Sea or Himalayan salt
- ☐ Asafoetida (optional)
- ☐ Ground cumin
- ☐ Dried oregano
- ☐ Ground ginger
- ☐ Ground turmeric
- ☐ Dried thyme
- ☐ Dried rosemary
- ☐ Dried parsley
- ☐ Dried dill
- ☐ Dried basil
- ☐ Vanilla extract

MEAL PREP FOR THE HEALING PHASE MEAL PLAN

GENERAL PREPARATION TIPS:

- **Plan Ahead:** Set aside time on the weekend to prep for the week ahead. Consider cooking larger batches of certain meals to save time during the week.
- **Storage:** Use clear, airtight containers to store prepped meals and ingredients. Label containers with the name and date for easy identification.
- **Batch Cooking:** Prepare larger portions of versatile ingredients (like grains, proteins, and vegetables) that can be used in multiple meals.
- **Cutting & Chopping:** Chop vegetables and fruits ahead of time, storing them in airtight containers in the fridge to keep them fresh.

SPECIFIC DAILY PREP TIPS:

Day 1:

- **Pumpkin Pancakes:** Prepare batter the night before and refrigerate. Cook in the morning.
- **Banana Avocado Smoothie:** Blend ingredients in the morning for a fresh taste.
- **Turkey Stroganoff:** Cook turkey and sauce in bulk, refrigerate, and reheat with roasted broccoli.
- **Baked Zucchini Fries:** Slice zucchini, coat in flour, and bake; store in the fridge for a quick snack.
- **Salmon Patties:** Prepare and cook salmon patties in advance; reheat before dinner.

Day 2:

- **French Toast:** Prep bread slices overnight; dip in egg mixture in the morning.
- **Pear Ginger Smoothie:** Blend fresh ingredients in the morning.
- **Sweet Potato Chicken Nuggets:** Cook in bulk and freeze extras for later.
- **Crispy Carrot Chips:** Bake in advance and store in an airtight container.
- **Butternut Squash Soup:** Make a large batch and refrigerate or freeze leftovers.

Day 3:

- **Sweet Potato Pancakes:** Prepare batter the night before; cook fresh in the morning.
- **Melon Smoothie:** Blend fresh ingredients in the morning.
- **Creamy Broccoli Potato Soup:** Make a big batch and reheat for lunch.
- **Pumpkin Donuts:** Bake in advance; store in a container to keep fresh.
- **Almond Crusted Chicken:** Prepare chicken and almond coating, bake when ready to eat.

Day 4:

- **Crustless Spinach Quiche:** Bake ahead of time; store in the fridge and reheat slices as needed.
- **Jasmine Milk Tea:** Brew in advance and refrigerate; serve chilled.
- **Chicken Ramen Bowl:** Prep broth and toppings in advance; cook noodles fresh before serving.
- **Broccoli Tots:** Bake and store in an airtight container for easy snacking.
- **Herb Shrimp Pasta:** Cook shrimp and pasta fresh; toss with herbs just before serving.

Day 5:

- **Zucchini Breakfast Bread:** Bake ahead and store for quick breakfasts.
- **Chicory Latte:** Brew fresh each morning for the best flavor.
- **Korean Rice Bowl:** Prepare rice and toppings in advance; assemble fresh at lunchtime.
- **Baked Yuca Fries:** Bake in bulk and store; reheat before eating.
- **Stuffed Cabbage Rolls:** Prepare and cook in advance; reheat for dinner.

Day 6:

- **Overnight Oats:** Prepare jars the night before for easy breakfasts.
- **Papaya Aloe Vera Smoothie:** Blend fresh in the morning.
- **Grilled Shrimp Skewers:** Prep and marinate shrimp in advance; grill fresh before serving.
- **Sweet Potato Brownies:** Bake ahead and store for snacks.
- **Creamy Macaroni Pasta:** Cook fresh pasta and sauce for dinner.

Day 7:

- **Pumpkin Waffles:** Prepare batter the night before; cook fresh in the morning.
- **Banana Mango Smoothie:** Blend fresh in the morning.
- **Creamy Chicken Kale Soup:** Make a large batch; reheat for lunch.
- **Gingerbread Cookies:** Bake in advance for a sweet afternoon snack.
- **Creamy Butternut Squash Pasta:** Cook fresh sauce and pasta for dinner.

Additional Tips:

- **Freezing:** Consider freezing meals like soups and stews for longer storage and convenience.
- **Reheating:** Use the stove or microwave to reheat meals, adding a splash of water to retain moisture.
- **Mix & Match:** Feel free to swap meals and snacks between days to suit your preferences.

Meal Plan for the Maintenance Phase

DAY 1

Breakfast	Quinoa Porridge (p. 48)
Mid-morning Snack	Date Energy Balls (p. 140)
Lunch	Chicken and Green Bean Stir-Fry (p. 72)
Afternoon Snack	Watermelon Cucumber Juice (p. 148)
Dinner	Baked Falafel with Creamed Spinach (p. 96, 119)

DAY 2

Breakfast	Mango Chia Pudding (p. 53)
Mid-morning Snack	Pumpkin Bread (p. 126)
Lunch	Turkey and Squash Rice Casserole (p. 78)
Afternoon Snack	Baked Yuca Fries (p. 141)
Dinner	Fish Tacos (p. 99)

DAY 3

Breakfast	Buckwheat Porridge (p. 58)
Mid-morning Snack	Date Energy Balls (p. 140)
Lunch	Crispy Sesame Tempeh (p. 81)
Afternoon Snack	Creamy Carob Mousse (p. 136)
Dinner	Butternut Squash Pasta (p. 104)

DAY 4

Breakfast	Blueberry Chia Pudding (p. 63)
Mid-morning Snack	Pumpkin Muffins (p. 133)
Lunch	Miso Soup (p. 93)
Afternoon Snack	Oatmeal Bars (p. 130)
Dinner	Lentil Meatballs (p. 87)

DAY 5	
Breakfast	Pumpkin Bread (p. 126)
Mid-morning Snack	Date Energy Balls (p. 140)
Lunch	Pecan Crusted Salmon (p. 90)
Afternoon Snack	Watermelon Cucumber Juice (p. 148)
Dinner	Fish Tacos (p. 99)

DAY 6	
Breakfast	Baked Oats (p. 52)
Mid-morning Snack	Pumpkin Muffins (p. 133)
Lunch	Crispy Sesame Tempeh (p. 81)
Afternoon Snack	Puffed Rice Bars (p. 138)
Dinner	Chicken Lentil Stew (p. 105)

DAY 7	
Breakfast	Blueberry Chia Pudding (p. 63)
Mid-morning Snack	Date Energy Balls (p. 140)
Lunch	Turkey Quinoa Meatloaf (p. 102)
Afternoon Snack	Oatmeal Bars (p. 130)
Dinner	Grilled Za'atar Chicken Tenders (p. 108)

SHOPPING LIST FOR THE MAINTENANCE PHASE MEAL PLAN

POULTRY AND EGGS

- ☐ 1½ pounds (about 680 g) lean ground chicken
- ☐ 2 pounds (about 900 g) lean ground turkey
- ☐ 1 pound (about 450 g) chicken tenderloins
- ☐ 9 large eggs

SEAFOOD

- ☐ 1 pound (about 450 g) white fish fillets (cod or tilapia)
- ☐ 2 salmon fillets (4 oz each)

PLANT-BASED PROTEINS

- ☐ 12 oz (about 340 g) firm tofu
- ☐ 8 oz (about 225 g) tempeh
- ☐ 1 small package dry chickpeas
- ☐ 1 small package dry lentils (black, green, or brown)
- ☐ 1 small package dry quinoa

PRODUCE

- ☐ 1 small watermelon (to yield at least 3 cups cubed)

- ☐ 1 English cucumber
- ☐ 16 Medjool dates
- ☐ 2 large mangoes
- ☐ 2 medium bananas
- ☐ 1 small container blueberries
- ☐ 2 leeks
- ☐ 2 medium carrots
- ☐ 1 bunch spinach, plus 1 bag baby spinach or kale
- ☐ 2 medium butternut squash (about 2½ pounds)
- ☐ 1 pound (about 450 g) green beans
- ☐ 2 large yucas (cassava)
- ☐ 3 ripe Hass avocados
- ☐ 1 lemon (for zest)
- ☐ 1 lime (optional, for zest)
- ☐ 1 small head purple cabbage
- ☐ 1 small head green cabbage
- ☐ 1 large bunch cilantro
- ☐ 1 small bunch parsley
- ☐ 1 small bunch thyme
- ☐ 8 sage leaves
- ☐ Small sprig rosemary
- ☐ Small piece ginger root

NUTS, SEEDS, AND GRAINS

- ☐ 1 (8 oz) package chia seeds
- ☐ 1 (4 oz) package coconut flakes
- ☐ 1 (8 oz) package unsweetened shredded coconut
- ☐ 1 (4 oz) package walnuts
- ☐ 1 (4 oz) package sliced almonds (optional)
- ☐ 1 (4 oz) package pecans, finely chopped
- ☐ 1 (16 oz) package buckwheat groats
- ☐ 1 (18 oz) package quick-cooking oats
- ☐ 1 (6 oz) box plain puffed rice cereal
- ☐ 1 (8 oz) tub white miso paste
- ☐ 1 (1 oz) package dried wakame
- ☐ 1 package package gluten-free tortillas (usually contains 6 or 8 tortillas)

OTHERS

- • 1 (22 oz) package gluten-free all-purpose flour
- • 1 liter coconut milk (carton-packed, not canned)
- • 1 liter unsweetened almond milk
- • 1 small container non-dairy plain yogurt (optional)
- • 1 small jar nut butter (no added sugars or oils)
- • 1 small container unsweetened applesauce (or 1 additional banana)

PANTRY ITEMS

- ☐ Maple syrup or honey
- ☐ Vanilla extract
- ☐ Olive oil
- ☐ Coconut oil (or avocado oil)
- ☐ Sesame oil
- ☐ Coconut aminos (or liquid aminos)
- ☐ Arrowroot flour (or potato starch)
- ☐ Baking powder
- ☐ Baking soda
- ☐ Xanthan gum (omit if your flour blend includes it)
- ☐ Carob powder
- ☐ Ground cumin
- ☐ Ground coriander
- ☐ Ground cinnamon
- ☐ Ground turmeric
- ☐ Ground ginger
- ☐ Ground nutmeg (optional)
- ☐ Sesame seeds
- ☐ Fennel seeds
- ☐ Sweet paprika (optional)
- ☐ Dried oregano
- ☐ Dried basil
- ☐ Dried rosemary
- ☐ Dried thyme
- ☐ Sumac
- ☐ Asafoetida powder (optional)
- ☐ Sea salt or Himalayan salt

MEAL PREP FOR THE MAINTENANCE PHASE MEAL PLAN

GENERAL PREPARATION TIPS:

- **Schedule Prep Time:** Designate a specific time each week (preferably on the weekend) to prepare as much as possible.
- **Container Strategy:** Use clear, labeled containers for different meals and snacks to keep everything organized and easily accessible.
- **Batch Cooking:** Prepare larger portions of base ingredients (grains, proteins, and vegetables) that can be used across multiple meals.
- **Prepping Ingredients:** Wash, chop, and portion out fruits and vegetables ahead of time to make assembly quick and easy.

SPECIFIC DAILY PREP TIPS:

Day 1:

- **Quinoa Porridge:** Cook quinoa in advance; reheat with milk or water and toppings in the morning.
- **Date Energy Balls:** Make a batch ahead of time; store in the fridge for easy snacking.
- **Chicken and Green Bean Stir-Fry**: Cook chicken and green beans in advance; reheat and serve fresh.
- **Watermelon Cucumber Juice:** Prepare fresh in the morning or the night before and store in the fridge.
- **Baked Falafel:** Prepare and bake falafel in advance; serve with creamed spinach that can be made ahead and reheated.

Day 2:

- **Mango Chia Pudding:** Prepare the night before; let chia seeds soak overnight.
- **Pumpkin Bread:** Bake in advance; store in an airtight container for fresh slices.
- **Turkey and Squash Rice Casserole:** Make a large batch and portion out for lunch.
- **Baked Yuca Fries:** Bake in advance and store; reheat as needed.
- **Fish Tacos:** Prepare fish fresh for dinner; have toppings ready in advance.

Day 3:

- **Buckwheat Porridge:** Cook buckwheat in advance; reheat with your choice of milk or toppings.
- **Date Energy Balls:** Make more if you're running low; store in the fridge.
- **Crispy Sesame Tempeh:** Prepare and cook tempeh ahead of time; reheat for lunch.
- **Creamy Carob Mousse:** Make in advance; store in the fridge for a refreshing snack.
- **Butternut Squash Risotto:** Cook fresh, or prepare ingredients (like roasted squash) ahead of time.

Day 4:

- **Blueberry Chia Pudding:** Prep the night before; let chia seeds soak overnight.
- **Pumpkin Muffins:** Bake ahead of time; store for easy mid-morning snacks.
- **Miso Soup:** Prepare broth and ingredients ahead; reheat for lunch.
- **Oatmeal Bars:** Make a batch in advance; store in an airtight container.
- **Lentil Meatballs:** Prepare and bake in advance; reheat for dinner.

Day 5:

- **Pumpkin Bread:** Use leftovers from Day 2 for breakfast.
- **Date Energy Balls:** Have a fresh batch ready for snacks.
- **Pecan Crusted Salmon:** Prepare salmon and crust ahead of time; bake fresh for lunch.
- **Watermelon Cucumber Juice:** Make fresh or batch prep the night before.
- **Fish Tacos:** Repeat from Day 2 for simplicity; have toppings prepped.

Day 6:

- **Baked Oats:** Prep and bake a batch ahead of time; reheat in the morning.
- **Pumpkin Muffins:** Use leftovers from Day 4 for a mid-morning snack.
- **Crispy Sesame Tempeh:** Cook extra if you have leftovers; store for lunch.
- **Puffed Rice Bars:** Make a batch ahead of time; store for snacking.
- **Chicken Lentil Stew:** Cook in bulk and store leftovers for easy reheating.

Day 7:

- **Blueberry Chia Pudding:** Use leftovers from Day 4 or prep fresh the night before.
- **Date Energy Balls:** Keep a fresh batch ready for snacks.
- **Turkey Quinoa Meatloaf:** Prepare and bake in advance; reheat for lunch.
- **Oatmeal Bars:** Use leftovers for an afternoon snack.
- **Grilled Za'atar Chicken Tenders:** Marinate and grill fresh for dinner.

Additional Tips:

- **Freezing:** Consider freezing extra servings of soups, casseroles, and baked goods for later use.
- **Reheating:** Use the stove or microwave to reheat meals, ensuring they are warmed through.
- **Mix & Match:** Feel free to swap snacks and meals between days to keep variety in your diet.

Tips for Buying Packaged Foods

The ingredients listed next are called for in many of the recipes. When purchasing, make sure they meet the following criteria:

- **GLUTEN-FREE BREAD** Avoid added vinegar and enzymes (making your own is recommended, see p. 162).

- **GLUTEN-FREE BREADCRUMBS** Unseasoned.

- **GLUTEN-FREE PASTA** Should be made from cassava flour, white rice, or sweet potato. Brown rice, though not entirely recommended, is acceptable in pasta form for most people.

- **GLUTEN-FREE FLOUR TORTILLAS** Can be made from cassava flour, sweet potatoes, cauliflower, almond flour, etc., depending on your preference and what you tolerate.

- **BAKING POWDER** Aluminum-free.

- **BROTHS (VEGETABLE OR CHICKEN)** Should not contain irritating ingredients such as onion and garlic.

- **PUFFED RICE CAKES** Prefer those made with white rice. If unavailable, puffed rice cakes made with brown rice are permissible during the first 90 days, as they are lighter and easier to digest.

- **ALMOND MILK** Preferably unsweetened and made with only three ingredients: water, almonds, and salt. This applies to other plant-based milks such as oat, coconut, and rice.

- **QUICK COOKING OR INSTANT OATS** Unflavored.

- **NUT BUTTERS** Should contain only two ingredients, e.g., almonds and salt, with no added sugars or oils.

- **CANNED COCONUT MILK** Should contain only water and coconut, without added gums or fibers.

- **COCONUT AMINOS** Avoid the one with added vinegar.

- **SHREDDED COCONUT** Unsweetened.

- **VANILLA EXTRACT** Preferably alcohol-free, especially when added to smoothies. If you must use extracts containing alcohol, note that much of the alcohol evaporates upon heating.

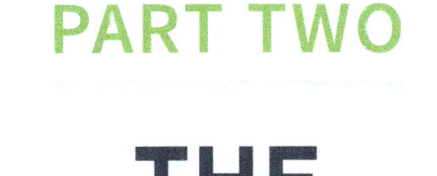

PART TWO

THE RECIPES

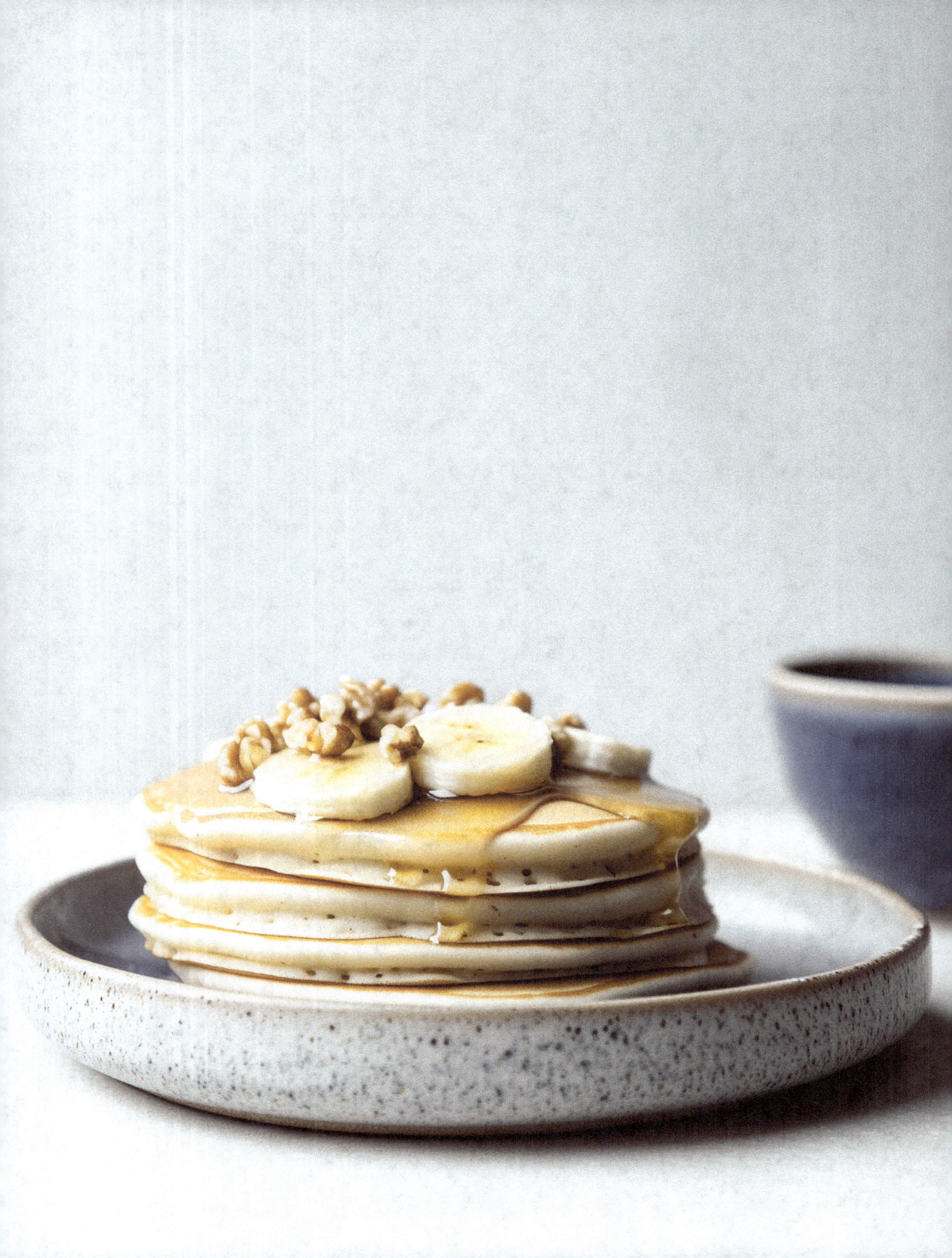

Chapter Four

BREAKFASTS

PUMPKIN PANCAKES

SERVES 4 pancakes

PREP 5 min

COOK 10 min

READY IN 15 min

INGREDIENTS

½ cup pumpkin purée (ensure it's not pumpkin pie filling)

½ cup gluten-free all-purpose flour (see note)

2 large eggs

½ teaspoon freshly grated ginger (optional, for a zesty twist)

DIRECTIONS

1. In a bowl, whisk together the beaten egg, egg white, pumpkin purée, gluten-free flour, and ginger until smooth.

2. Preheat a nonstick skillet over medium-high heat and lightly grease it with coconut oil or cooking spray.

3. Scoop about ¼ cup of batter for each pancake onto the hot skillet, spreading slightly if needed.

4. Cook the pancakes until bubbles form on the surface and the edges are set, about 2-3 minutes. Check for a golden brown underside.

5. Flip the pancakes and cook for an additional 3 minutes, or until the other side is also golden brown and the pancakes are cooked through.

NOTE

- For an alternative to gluten-free all-purpose flour, you can use an equivalent amount of gluten-free pancake mix or oat flour for a slightly different texture.

PER SERVING (2 pancakes)
Calories: 178; Total fat: 3g; Protein: 6g;
Carbohydrates: 27g; Fiber: 2g

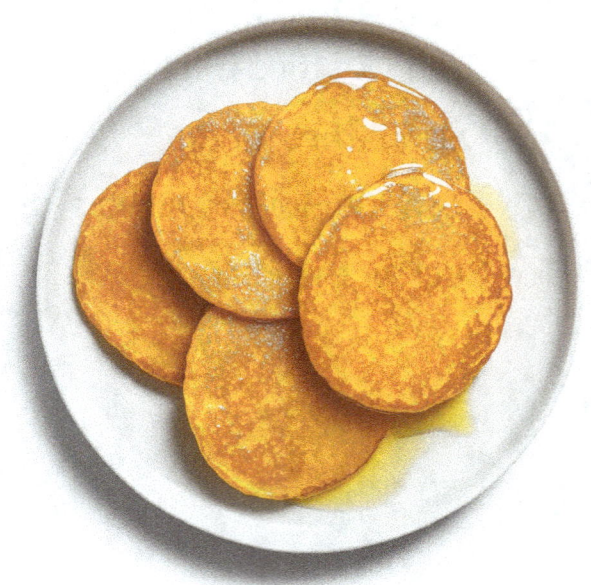

OVERNIGHT OATS

SERVES 1

PREP 5 min

COOK n/a

READY IN 4-8 hours

INGREDIENTS

½ cup quick-cooking or unflavored instant oats

½ cup almond milk (or other plant-based milk)

1 tablespoon maple syrup

1 teaspoon chia seeds (optional, for maintenance phase)

Toppings: ½ sliced banana and 1 tablespoon chopped walnuts (see note)

DIRECTIONS

1. In a small jar, combine the oats, almond milk, maple syrup, and chia seeds (if using).

2. Secure the jar with a lid or cover tightly with plastic wrap. Refrigerate for at least 4 hours or overnight.

3. Before serving, stir the oats and adjust the consistency by adding more milk if desired. Add toppings either before chilling or just before serving.

4. Serve chilled and enjoy!

NOTE

- Feel free to customize the toppings based on your preferences and tolerances. The banana and walnuts add a nice texture and are packed with nutrients. However, other toppings like Bosc pear, coconut flakes, or nut butter can also be used to vary the flavor and nutritional content.

PER SERVING (about 1 cup) Calories: 339; Total fat: 9g; Protein: 8g; Carbohydrates: 50g; Fiber: 7g

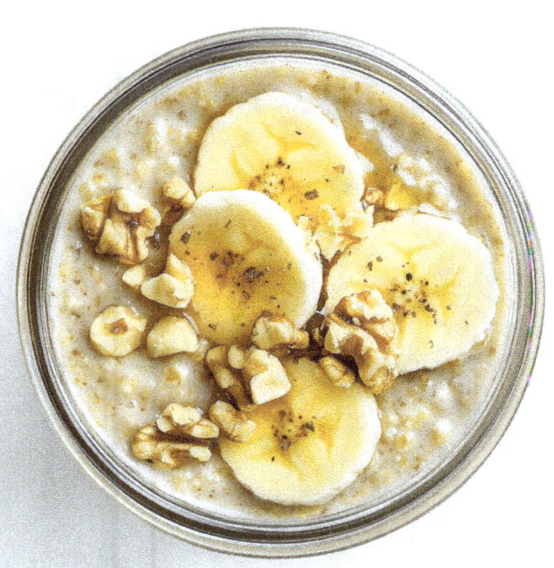

STUFFED SWEET POTATO

SERVES 1

PREP 5 min

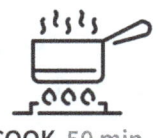
COOK 50 min

READY IN 55 min

INGREDIENTS

1 medium sweet potatoes

1 whole egg

1 egg white

¼ cup mashed avocado

Salt to taste

Fresh cilantro, chopped
(optional, for garnish)

DIRECTIONS

1. Preheat the oven to 400 degrees Fahrenheit. Wash and poke holes in the sweet potato. Place on a parchment-lined baking sheet and bake for 45-55 minutes, until tender.

2. In a small bowl, whisk the eggs with salt to taste.

3. Heat a non-stick skillet over medium-low heat. Once hot, pour the whisked eggs into the skillet. Scramble the eggs, stirring continuously with a silicone or wooden spatula, until they reach your desired consistency.

4. Split the baked sweet potato lengthwise, gently open to make room, and fill with scrambled eggs and mashed avocado. Sprinkle chopped fresh cilantro on top before serving for a fresh, herby finish.

PER SERVING (1 stuffed sweet potato)
Calories: 264; Total fat: 10g; Protein: 13g; Carbohydrates: 20g; Fiber: 7g

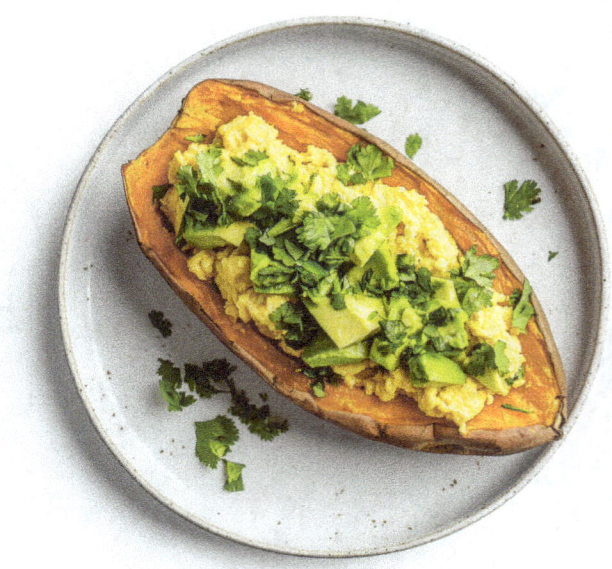

PUMPKIN WAFFLES

SERVES 4 waffles

PREP 10 min

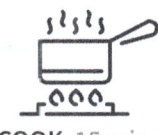

COOK 15 min

READY IN 25 min

INGREDIENTS

1 (15 oz.) can pumpkin purée (not pumpkin pie filling)

1 ¼ cups gluten-free all-purpose flour

½ teaspoon xanthan gum (omit if your flour includes it)

2 egg whites

¼ cup maple syrup or honey

½ cup unsweetened almond milk

2 tablespoons olive oil

1 teaspoon baking powder

1 teaspoon vanilla extract

½ teaspoon salt

½ teaspoon ground cinnamon (optional, for maintenance phase)

DIRECTIONS

1. In a large mixing bowl, combine pumpkin purée, egg whites, olive oil, vanilla extract, maple syrup or honey, and salt. Mix until smooth.

2. Stir in the gluten-free flour, baking powder, xanthan gum (if using), and cinnamon until just combined. Gradually add the almond milk to reach a thick batter consistency.

3. Preheat your waffle iron and coat with gluten-free cooking spray.

4. Pour ⅓ cup of batter into the waffle iron for each waffle, using an ice cream scoop for even distribution.

5. Cook according to your waffle iron's instructions until the waffles are golden and crisp.

NOTE

- Leftover waffles can be stored in an airtight container in the fridge for up to 3 days. Reheat in a toaster or oven for best results.

PER SERVING (1 waffle) Calories: 298; Total fat: 8g; Protein: 3g; Carbohydrates: 48g; Fiber: 3g

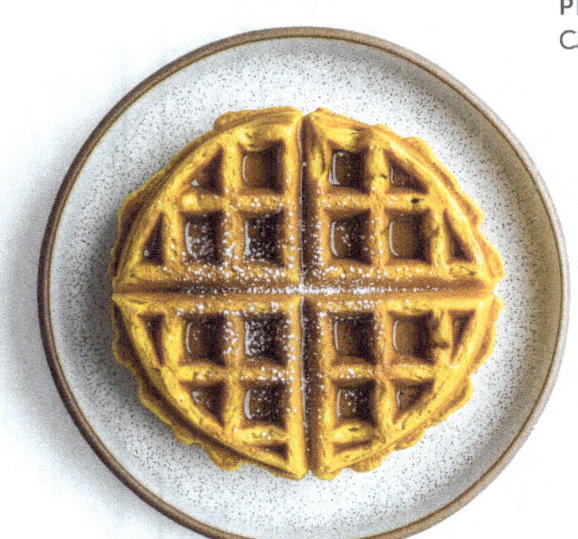

QUINOA PORRIDGE

SERVES 2

PREP 10 min

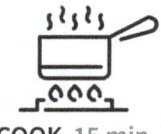
COOK 15 min

READY IN 25 min

INGREDIENTS

½ cup uncooked quinoa

2 ¼ cups coconut milk (carton-packed, not canned)

1-2 tablespoons maple syrup

1 teaspoon vanilla extract

2 tablespoons coconut flakes

2 tablespoons sliced almonds (optional)

DIRECTIONS

1. Rinse the quinoa thoroughly and drain.

2. In a medium saucepan, combine the rinsed quinoa, coconut milk, maple syrup, and vanilla extract. Bring to a boil over medium-high heat.

3. Once boiling, reduce the heat to low and let it simmer for 15 minutes, or until most of the liquid is absorbed and the quinoa is tender.

4. Divide the porridge evenly between two bowls. Stir in a little more milk if needed to reach your desired creaminess.

5. Top with coconut flakes or sliced almonds if using. Serve warm and enjoy!

PER SERVING (about 1 ¼ cups)
Calories: 264; Total fat: 10g; Protein: 6g;
Carbohydrates: 32g; Fiber: 5g

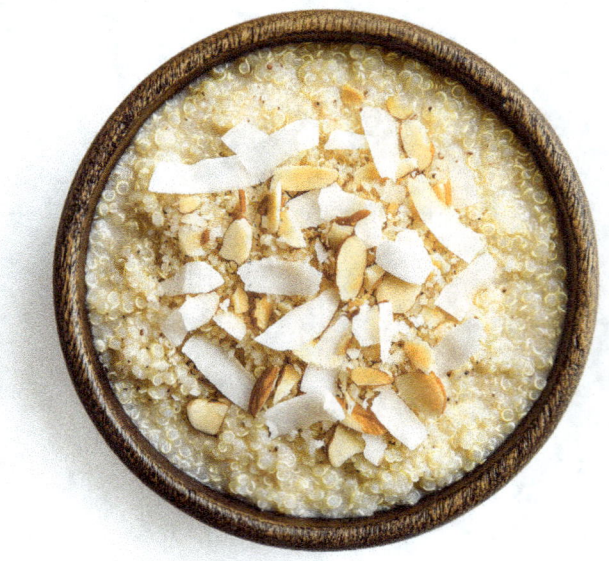

TURKEY BREAKFAST SAUSAGE

SERVES 4 patties

PREP 10 min

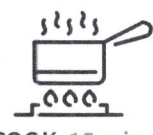
COOK 15 min

READY IN 25 min

INGREDIENTS

½ pound lean ground turkey (about 1 cup)

2 teaspoons ground sage

½ teaspoon dried thyme

1 tablespoon olive oil

½ teaspoon salt

DIRECTIONS

1. In a medium bowl, mix the ground turkey with sage, thyme, and salt until well combined.

2. Form the mixture into about 4 patties.

3. Heat oil in a large nonstick skillet over medium-high heat. Once the oil shimmers, add the patties.

4. Cook the patties for about 4 minutes per side, or until they are browned and cooked through.

5. Transfer the patties to a paper towel-lined plate to drain any excess oil. Serve and enjoy!

NOTE

- To make ahead, double the batch and freeze. Wrap each patty individually in plastic wrap and place in a ziplock or resealable freezer bag. Store in the freezer for up to 3 months.

PER SERVING (1 patty) Calories: 120; Total fat: 6.5g; Protein: 15g; Carbohydrates: 0g; Fiber: 0g

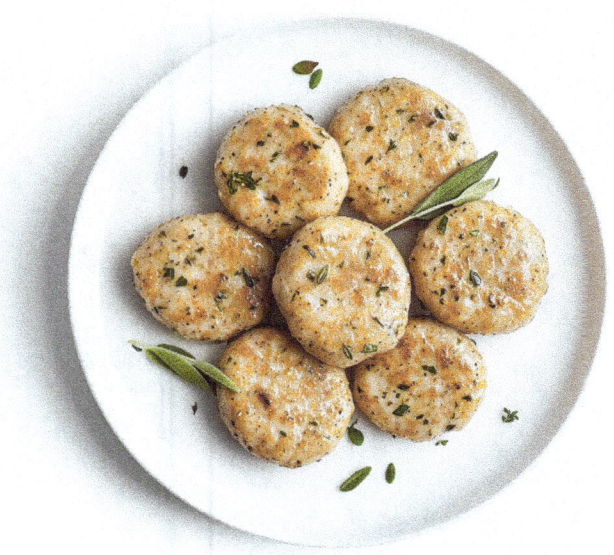

SWEET POTATO PANCAKES

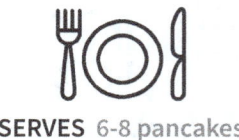
SERVES 6-8 pancakes

PREP 10 min

COOK 15 min

READY IN 25 min

INGREDIENTS

1 cup mashed sweet potato (see notes)

2 large eggs

½ cup unsweetened almond milk

¾ cup gluten-free all-purpose flour (see notes)

2-3 tablespoons maple syrup

1 tablespoon olive oil

1 teaspoon baking powder

¼ teaspoon salt

½ teaspoon cinnamon powder (optional, for maintenance phase)

DIRECTIONS

1. In a bowl, combine mashed sweet potato, eggs, almond milk, and maple syrup. Whisk until well blended.

2. Over the sweet potato mixture, evenly sprinkle flour, baking powder, salt, and cinnamon (if using). Stir until the batter is smooth.

3. Heat the oil in a large nonstick skillet over medium heat. Once hot, pour ⅓ cup portions of batter onto the skillet. Cook until bubbles appear on the surface of the pancakes, about 2-4 minutes.

4. Flip the pancakes and cook for another 2-3 minutes until golden and cooked through.

5. Repeat with the remaining batter, making approximately 6-8 pancakes.

6. Serve the pancakes warm, topped with additional maple syrup.

NOTES

- To make mashed sweet potato, bake or boil peeled sweet potatoes until tender, then mash until smooth.

- You can substitute the gluten-free flour with oat flour or another preferred gluten-free blend.

PER SERVING (2 pancakes)
Calories: 220; Total fat: 4g; Protein: 4g;
Carbohydrates: 34g; Fiber: 2g

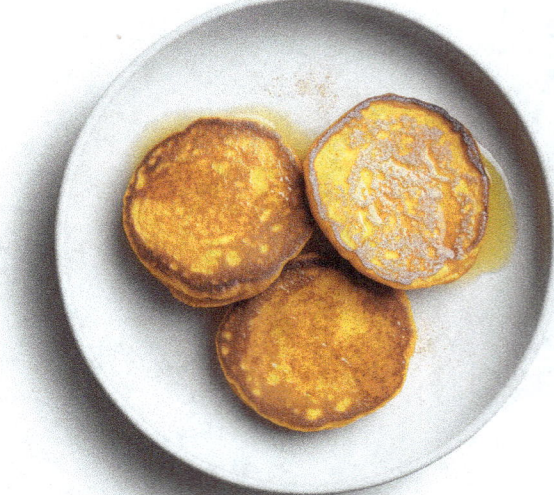

SPANISH OMELETTE

 **SERVES** 4

 **PREP** 10 min

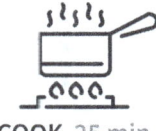 **COOK** 25 min

 **READY IN** 35 min

INGREDIENTS

1 pound potatoes, peeled and diced (about 1⅔ cups)

½ cup leek (white part only), diced

3 large eggs, lightly beaten

3 egg whites, lightly beaten

1 tablespoon olive oil

2 tablespoons fresh parsley, finely chopped

2 tablespoons fresh basil, finely chopped

Salt to taste

Fresh herb sprigs (optional, for garnish)

DIRECTIONS

1. In a large pan, cover the potatoes with water and bring to a boil. Cook uncovered for 3 minutes. Remove from heat, cover, and let stand for about 10 minutes or until the potatoes are tender. Drain well.

2. Heat the oil in a deep, 10-inch nonstick skillet over medium heat. Add the diced leek and cook for about 8 minutes, stirring occasionally.

3. Add the drained potatoes to the skillet and continue to cook for 5 more minutes.

4. In a bowl, combine the whole eggs, egg whites, parsley, and basil. Season with salt.

5. Pour the egg mixture over the potatoes in the skillet. Reduce the heat and cook uncovered for about 10 minutes, or until the bottom of the omelet is golden and set.

6. Optionally, brown the top under a broiler or in a toaster oven for a few minutes.

7. Garnish with fresh herb sprigs if using, and serve.

PER SERVING (¼ of the omelette) Calories 168; Total fat 7g; Protein: 10g; Carbohydrates: 12g; Fiber: 2g

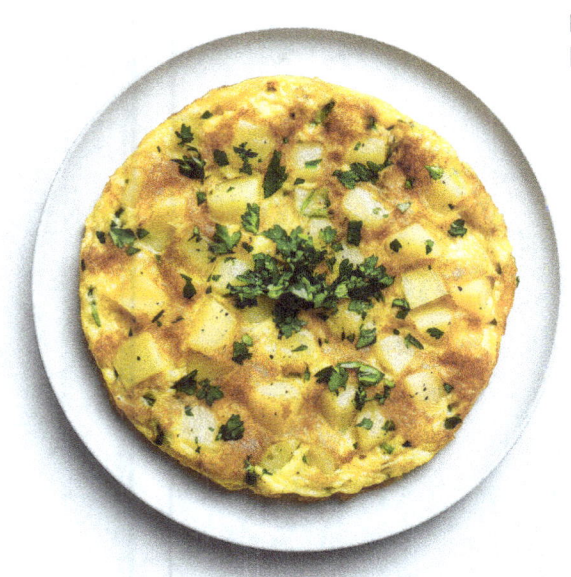

BAKED OATS

 **SERVES** 2

 **PREP** 5 min

 **COOK** 30 min

 **READY IN** 35 min

INGREDIENTS

1 cup quick-cooking oats

½ cup unsweetened almond milk

1 medium banana

1 large egg

2 tablespoons maple syrup or honey

1 teaspoon baking powder

1 teaspoon vanilla extract

1 teaspoon cinnamon powder (optional, for maintenance phase)

Pinch of salt

DIRECTIONS

1. Preheat your oven to 375°F (190°C).

2. In a blender, combine oats, almond milk, banana, egg, maple syrup or honey, baking powder, vanilla extract, cinnamon (if using), and a pinch of salt. Blend for about 1 minute until smooth.

3. Pour the batter into 2-3 small ramekins, or double the batch for a large 9x13-inch casserole dish.

4. Bake in the preheated oven for 30 minutes, or until the oats are set and lightly golden on top.

5. Remove from the oven and, if desired, drizzle with additional maple syrup. Serve warm and enjoy!

PER SERVING (about 1 cup)
Calories: 305; Total fat: 6g; Protein: 9g;
Carbohydrates: 49g; Fiber: 5g

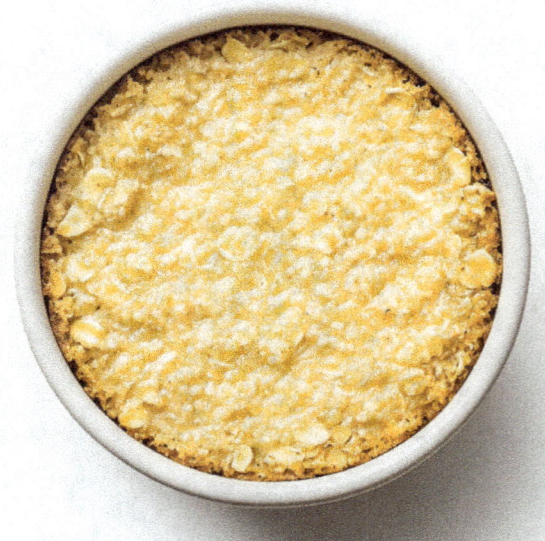

MANGO CHIA PUDDING

SERVES 2

PREP 5 min

COOK n/a

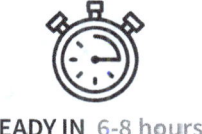

READY IN 6-8 hours

INGREDIENTS

1 large mango, peeled and sliced

1 cup unsweetened almond milk

2-3 tablespoons maple syrup or honey

¼ cup chia seeds

Optional for topping: additional chopped mango, coconut flakes

DIRECTIONS

1. In a blender or food processor, combine the mango slices and ½ cup of the almond milk. Process until a smooth purée forms.

2. Pour the mango purée into a large bowl. Add the remaining ½ cup almond milk, maple syrup (or honey), and chia seeds, if using.

3. Mix well using a spoon or fork, then let the mixture sit for about 10 minutes. Stir again to ensure even distribution of the chia seeds.

4. Cover the bowl and refrigerate overnight, or for at least 6 hours, allowing the chia seeds to absorb the liquid and thicken the pudding.

5. Before serving, stir the pudding once more. If desired, top with additional chopped mango and coconut flakes for extra flavor and texture.

PER SERVING (about ¾ cup) Calories: 267; Total fat: 8g; Protein 5g; Carbohydrates: 37g; Fiber: 9g

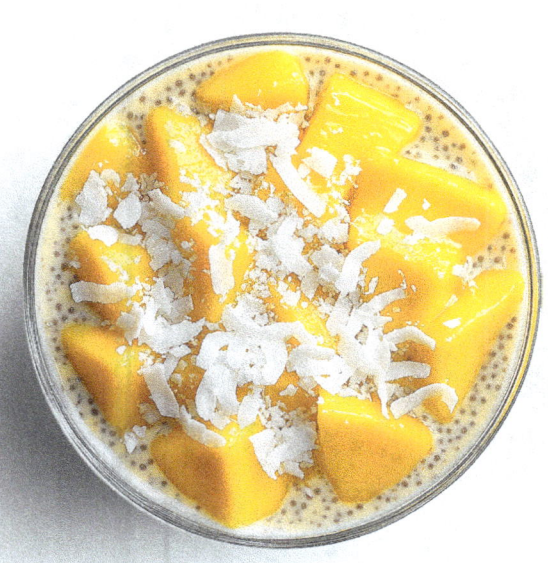

FRENCH TOAST

SERVES 2

PREP 10 min

COOK 10 min

READY IN 20 min

INGREDIENTS

1 large egg, beaten

1 egg white

½ cup almond milk

½ teaspoon vanilla extract

4 slices gluten-free bread

Pinch of salt

¼ teaspoon cinnamon powder
(optional, for maintenance
phase)

DIRECTIONS

1. In a medium bowl, whisk together the beaten egg, egg white, almond milk, vanilla extract, salt, and cinnamon (if using) until well combined.

2. Pour the egg mixture into a shallow dish. Soak each slice of bread in the mixture for about 3 minutes per side, ensuring they are thoroughly saturated but not falling apart.

3. Heat a large nonstick skillet over medium-high heat and grease it with coconut oil or non-stick cooking spray.

4. Place the soaked bread slices in the skillet. Cook for 3 to 4 minutes on each side or until the bread is golden brown and the custard is set.

5. Serve the French toast warm, topped with maple syrup or your choice of toppings.

PER SERVING (2 slices) Calories: 205;
Total fat: 7g; Protein: 6g; Carbohydrates:
27g; Fiber: 1g

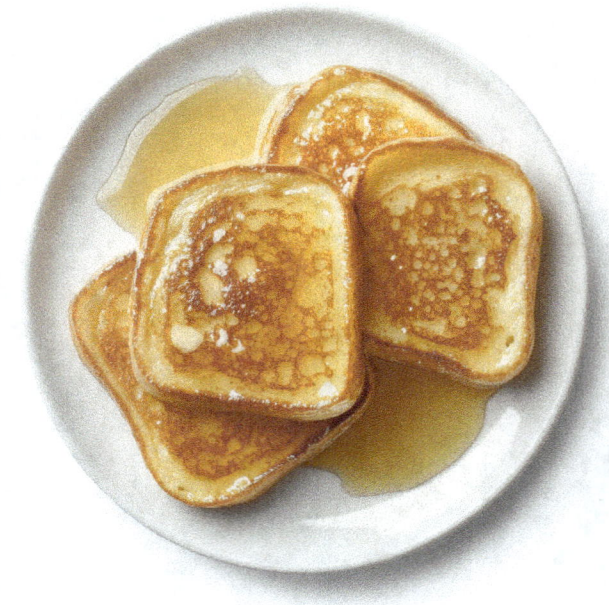

CREAM OF RICE CEREAL

SERVES 2

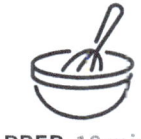
PREP 10 min

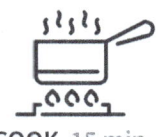
COOK 15 min

READY IN 25 min

INGREDIENTS

½ cup uncooked white rice

2 ¼ cups almond milk

Pinch of salt

Optional toppings: banana slices, coconut flakes, chopped walnuts, maple syrup

DIRECTIONS

1. Using a blender or coffee grinder, coarsely grind the white rice.

2. Pour the almond milk into a medium saucepan and bring it to a low boil over medium heat, stirring constantly to prevent it from burning.

3. Stir in the coarsely ground rice and a pinch of salt. Reduce the heat to low.

4. Cover the saucepan and let it simmer for 5 to 15 minutes, or until the mixture has thickened to your desired consistency, stirring occasionally. Monitor the mixture closely and add more almond milk as needed to prevent the rice from sticking to the bottom of the pan.

5. Serve the cream of rice warm, topped with your choice of banana slices, coconut flakes, chopped walnuts, or a drizzle of maple syrup

PER SERVING (about 1 cup) Calories: 234; Total fat: 3g; Protein 4g; Carbohydrates: 44g; Fiber: 2g

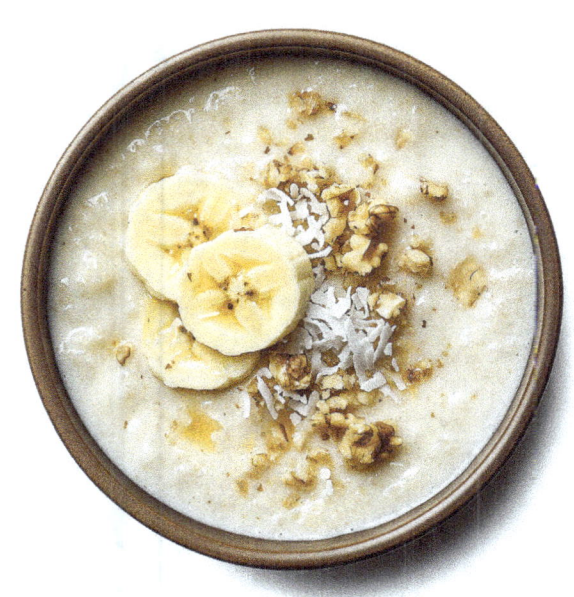

OAT WAFFLES

SERVES 4 waffles

PREP 10 min

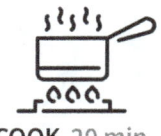

COOK 20 min

READY IN 30 min

INGREDIENTS

2 cups oat flour

1 cup unsweetened almond milk

1 large egg

2 large egg whites

1 tablespoon maple syrup or honey

2 teaspoons baking powder

1 teaspoon vanilla extract

Coconut oil for greasing

Optional toppings: maple syrup, almond butter, and/or fruits with a pH higher than 5

DIRECTIONS

1. In a blender, combine oat flour, almond milk, whole egg, egg whites, baking powder, maple syrup, and vanilla. Blend until smooth. Let the batter rest and thicken for about 10 minutes.

2. Preheat the waffle iron and grease each side with ½ teaspoon of coconut oil or non-stick cooking spray.

3. Pour about ¾ cup of the batter onto the heated waffle iron and close the lid. Cook for 6 to 8 minutes or until the waffle is golden brown.

4. Remove the waffle and place it on a plate or in an oven at 200°C to keep warm. Repeat with the remaining batter, greasing the waffle iron each time.

5. Serve immediately with your favorite toppings.

NOTE

- Store the remaining waffles between parchment paper in the fridge for up to 4 days or freeze for up to 2 months. For best results, reheat waffles in a toaster oven.

PER SERVING (1 waffle) Calories: 277; Total fat: 6g; Protein: 11g; Carbohydrates: 38g; Fiber: 6g

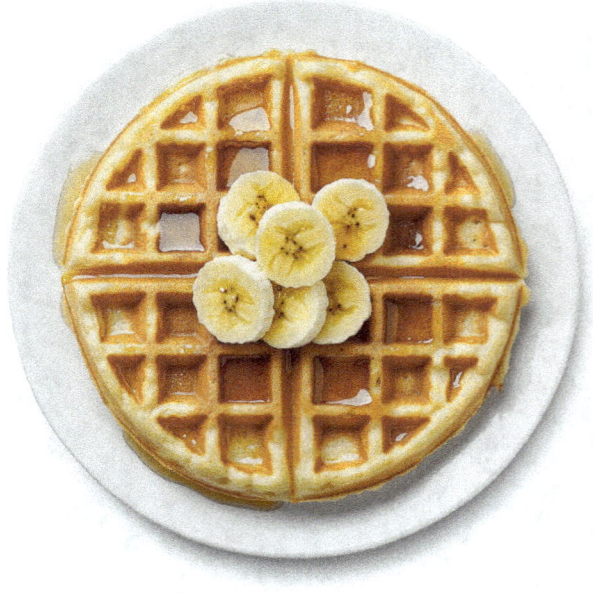

COCONUT FLOUR PANCAKES

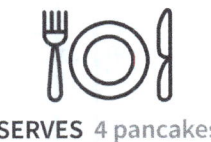
SERVES 4 pancakes

PREP 5 min

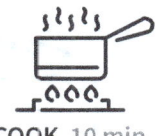
COOK 10 min

READY IN 15 min

INGREDIENTS

⅓ cup coconut flour

2 egg whites

1 large egg

2 tablespoons unsweetened almond milk

1 tablespoon coconut oil, melted

½ teaspoon baking powder

¼ teaspoon baking soda

1 tablespoon maple syrup or honey

1 teaspoon pure vanilla extract

Pinch of salt

DIRECTIONS

1. In a large bowl, combine coconut flour, baking powder, baking soda, and salt.

2. In another bowl, whisk eggs, almond milk, melted coconut oil, maple syrup, and vanilla extract until well blended.

3. Gradually mix the dry ingredients into the wet ingredients, stirring until just combined to avoid tough pancakes.

4. Heat a lightly greased skillet over medium heat. Scoop about ¼ cup of batter per pancake onto the skillet.

5. Cook each pancake for 2-3 minutes per side, or until golden brown and cooked through. Check for doneness by gently lifting one edge of the pancake.

6. Repeat with remaining batter, greasing the skillet as needed between batches.

7. Serve warm with your favorite toppings.

NOTES

- Let the batter rest for about 5 minutes before cooking to enhance fluffiness.

- If the batter is too thick, add a bit more milk or water to achieve a pourable consistency.

- Store pancakes in an airtight container in the refrigerator for up to three days or freeze them for up to three months with parchment paper between each pancake.

PER SERVING (1 pancake) Calories: 112; Total fat: 5g; Protein: 5g; Carbohydrates: 6g; Fiber: 3g

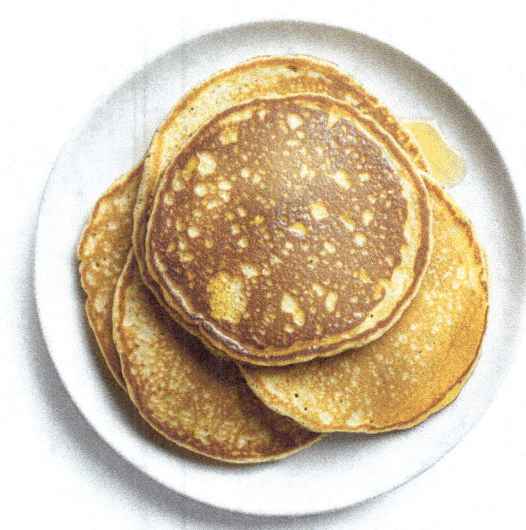

BUCKWHEAT PORRIDGE

 **SERVES** 1    **PREP** 15 min   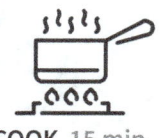 **COOK** 15 min    **READY IN** 30 min

INGREDIENTS

½ cup buckwheat groats, soaked and drained (see note)

½ cup unsweetened almond milk

¼ cup water

1 teaspoon vanilla extract

1-2 tablespoons maple syrup

Dash of cinnamon powder (optional)

DIRECTIONS

1. In a non-stick saucepan, combine the water, almond milk, and maple syrup. If using, whisk in protein powder until fully incorporated. Bring the mixture to a boil over medium heat.

2. Add the buckwheat groats, stir, then cover with a lid. Reduce the heat to a simmer and cook for 8-10 minutes, stirring occasionally, until all the liquid is absorbed. It's normal for a brown layer to form on the top; this does not affect the flavor.

3. Remove the saucepan from the heat. Stir in vanilla and, if desired, cinnamon. Cover and let sit for 5 minutes to allow the flavors to meld.

4. Uncover and fluff the porridge with a fork before serving. Enjoy warm.

NOTE

• To soak buckwheat groats, place them in a bowl of water for a few hours or overnight; this helps to soften them and reduce cooking time. Drain and rinse well before using.

PER SERVING (about 1 cup)
Calories: 353; Total fat: 3g; Protein: 10g; Carbohydrates: 66g; Fiber: 8g

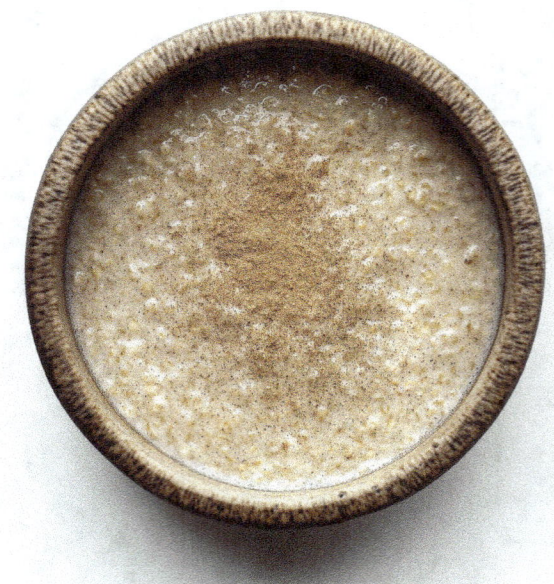

STEWED FRUIT MEDLEY

 **SERVES** 2

 **PREP** 10 min

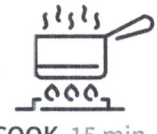 **COOK** 15 min

 **READY IN** 25 min

INGREDIENTS

1 banana, sliced

1 cup cantaloupe, cubed

1 Asian pear, cored and sliced

1 cup watermelon, cubed

1 dragon fruit, peeled and cubed

¼ cup water

2 tablespoons maple syrup (optional, for added sweetness)

½ teaspoon cinnamon powder (optional, for maintenance phase)

DIRECTIONS

1. In a medium saucepan, combine the fruits with water, maple syrup, and cinnamon if using.

2. Place the pan over medium heat and bring the mixture to a gentle simmer, stirring occasionally.

3. Allow the fruits to simmer for 10-15 minutes until they are tender but still have some texture.

4. Remove from heat and let the stewed fruits cool slightly before serving.

5. Serve warm or refrigerate to chill for a cool treat. This dish is great as a topping for oatmeal or enjoyed on its own as a light breakfast.

NOTE

- Any leftovers can be stored in an airtight container in the refrigerator for up to 3 days. Enjoy chilled or gently reheated.

PER SERVING (about 1½ cups) Calories: 136; Total fat: 0g; Protein: 2g; Carbohydrates: 27g; Fiber: 5g

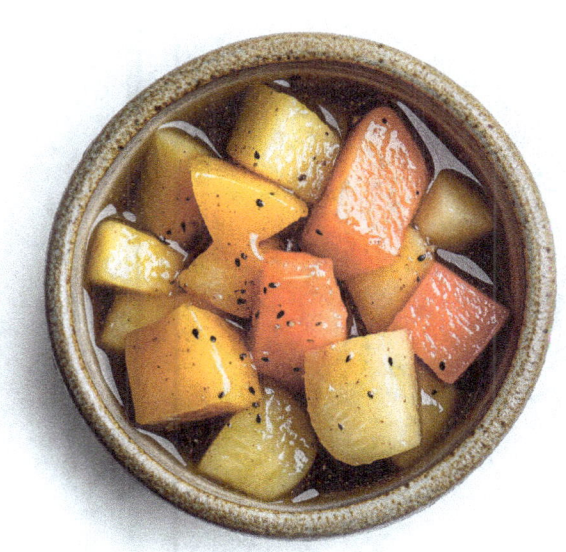

CRUSTLESS SPINACH QUICHE

   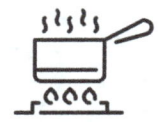 

SERVES 4   **PREP** 15 min   **COOK** 35 min   **READY IN** 50 min

INGREDIENTS

1 leek (white part only), diced

6 cups fresh spinach, roughly chopped

2 tablespoons olive oil

2 whole eggs, beaten

2 egg whites

1 ½ cups unsweetened almond milk

1 teaspoon dried parsley

1 teaspoon salt

¼ teaspoon asafoetida (optional)

DIRECTIONS

1. Preheat the oven to 400°F. Heat olive oil in a 12-inch cast iron skillet over medium-high heat, then add the diced leeks and sauté for about 5 minutes until translucent.

2. Add the fresh spinach to the skillet and cook for another 2 minutes until it wilts, then sprinkle with salt and asafoetida, mixing well.

3. In a medium bowl, whisk together the eggs and almond milk. Pour this mixture over the sautéed spinach and leeks in the skillet, stirring until all ingredients are evenly distributed.

4. Transfer the skillet to the middle rack of the oven and bake for 25 to 30 minutes, or until the quiche is firm to the touch.

5. Allow the quiche to cool, then store it in an airtight container in the refrigerator for up to 5 days.

NOTES

- If you don't have a cast iron skillet, you can sauté the ingredients in a regular skillet and then transfer them to an oven-proof casserole dish or pie pan for baking.

PER SERVING (¼ of the quiche)
Calories: 135; Total fat: 10g; Protein: 6g; Carbohydrates: 4g; Fiber: 1g

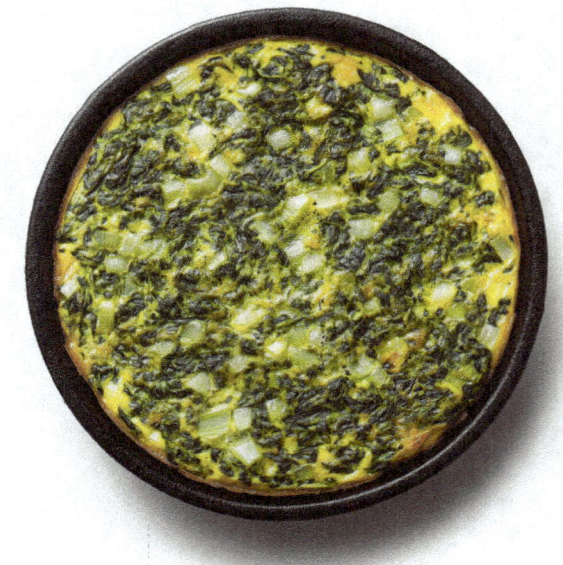

ZUCCHINI BREAKFAST BREAD

SERVES 10 slices

PREP 15 min

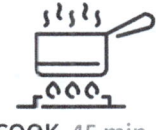
COOK 45 min

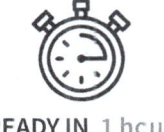
READY IN 1 hour

INGREDIENTS

1 medium zucchini

2 large eggs

1 ½ cups gluten-free all-purpose flour (make sure it contains xanthan gum)

¼ cup olive oil

½ cup maple syrup or honey

½ teaspoon baking soda

½ teaspoon baking powder

½ teaspoon dried or fresh lemon zest

1 teaspoon vanilla extract

½ teaspoon salt

1 tablespoon ground cinnamon (optional, for maintenance phase)

DIRECTIONS

1. Preheat the oven to 350°F (177°C).

2. Grease a 4x8-inch loaf pan with gluten-free cooking spray; a glass pan is recommended for even baking.

3. Shred the zucchini using a grater to yield 1 cup of shredded zucchini; keep the skin on and retain the moisture.

4. In a large mixing bowl, whisk together the eggs, olive oil, maple syrup (or honey), and vanilla extract until well combined.

5. Add salt, baking soda, baking powder, lemon zest, and cinnamon (if using) to the bowl. Mix these into the wet ingredients before folding in the gluten-free flour to ensure even distribution.

6. Stir the shredded zucchini into the batter until everything is well combined.

7. Transfer the batter to the prepared loaf pan, spreading it evenly.

8. Bake in the center of the oven for 45-55 minutes, or until a toothpick inserted into the center of the bread comes out clean. Keep an eye on the bread as it bakes, as oven temperatures can vary.

9. Allow the bread to cool in the pan before transferring it to a wire rack to cool completely.

10. Slice and serve. Store any leftovers in an airtight container at room temperature for 1-2 days or refrigerate for up to a week.

PER SERVING (1 slice) Calories: 172; Total fat: 6g; Protein: 2g; Carbohydrates: 25g; Fiber: 1g

BANANA AVOCADO SMOOTHIE

 **SERVES** 1

 **PREP** 5 min

 **COOK** n/a

 **READY IN** 7 min

INGREDIENTS

1 ripe banana

¼ cup mashed avocado

1 ½ cups almond milk

1 tablespoon maple syrup

½ teaspoon fresh ginger, grated
(optional)

DIRECTIONS

1. Place all the ingredients in a blender and blend until smooth.

2. Serve immediately and enjoy!

PER SERVING (about 2 cups)
Calories: 280; Total fat: 9g; Protein: 4g;
Carbohydrates: 42g; Fiber: 7g

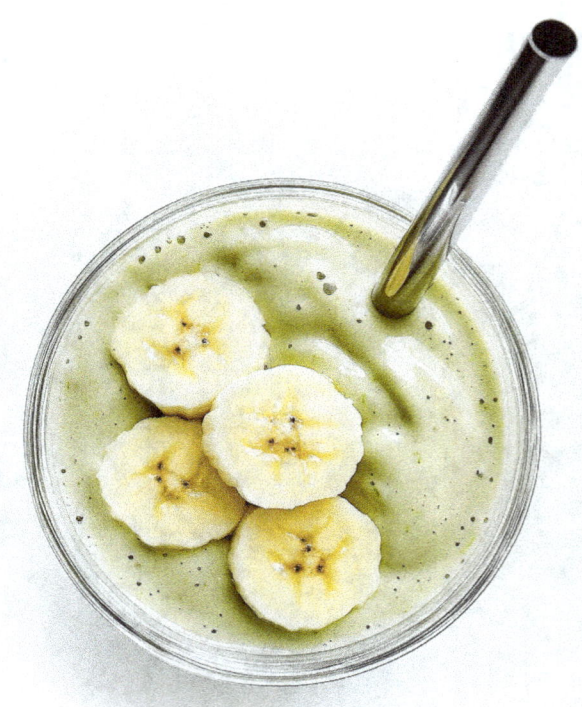

BLUEBERRY CHIA PUDDING

SERVES 1

PREP 10 min

COOK n/a

READY IN 2 hours

INGREDIENTS

½ cup almond milk

¼ cup fresh blueberries

2 tablespoons chia seeds

1 tablespoon maple syrup or honey

½ teaspoon vanilla extract (optional)

DIRECTIONS

1. Combine the almond milk and blueberries in a blender. Blend until smooth.

2. Pour the blueberry-almond milk mixture into a sealable jar or a bowl. Stir in the chia seeds, maple syrup, and vanilla extract, if using. Mix thoroughly to combine.

3. Let the mixture sit for about 10 minutes, then stir again to ensure there are no clumps.

4. Refrigerate the pudding for at least 2 hours, though leaving it overnight will yield the best results.

5. Before serving, give the pudding another stir to mix well. Serve chilled, drizzled with of maple syrup and other toppings of your choice.

PER SERVING (about 1 cup) Calories: 198; Total fat: 7g; Protein: 4g; Carbohydrates: 23g; Fiber: 8g

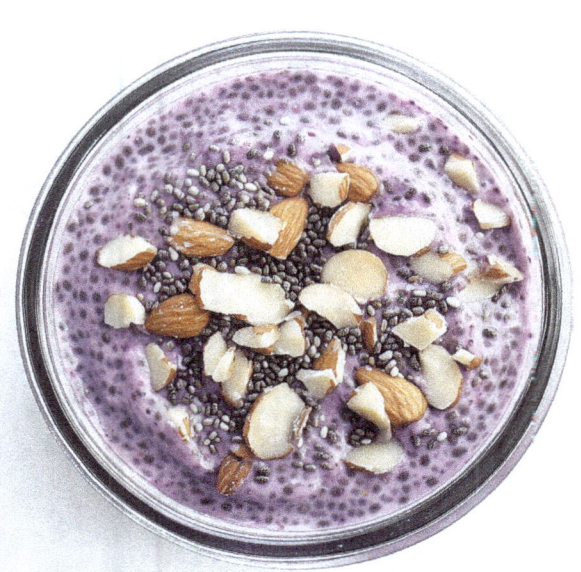

PUMPKIN HARVEST HASH

  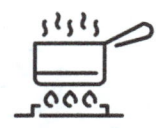 

SERVES 2   **PREP** 25 min   **COOK** 25 min   **READY IN** 50 min

INGREDIENTS

½ pound lean ground turkey (about 1 cup)

½ cup pumpkin, cubed

1 cup kale, chopped

1 cup mushrooms, diced

2 tablespoons chicken or vegetable broth (optional)

½ teaspoon dried oregano

½ teaspoon asafoetida (optional)

1 tablespoon olive oil

½ teaspoon salt

1 sprig fresh thyme

2 teaspoons fresh sage, chopped

DIRECTIONS

1. In a small bowl, mix the salt, oregano, and asafoetida (if using) to make the seasoning mixture.

2. Heat a medium skillet over medium heat. Add the ground turkey and the prepared seasoning mixture. Cook until the turkey is browned, stirring occasionally to crumble. Remove the turkey from the skillet and set aside.

3. In the same skillet, add the olive oil followed by the diced mushrooms and leaves from the fresh thyme sprig. Cook for about 2 minutes, stirring occasionally.

4. Add the cubed pumpkin to the skillet, season with a bit more salt, and cook, stirring occasionally, until the pumpkin is tender.

5. Return the browned turkey to the skillet. Add the broth (if using) and fresh sage. Reduce heat to a simmer and cook for an additional 2 to 3 minutes.

6. Stir in the chopped kale and cook just until the kale is wilted.

7. Serve warm and enjoy the hearty flavors of the harvest.

PER SERVING (about 1 cup)
Calories: 162; Total fat: 9g; Protein: 17g; Carbohydrates: 3g; Fiber: 2g

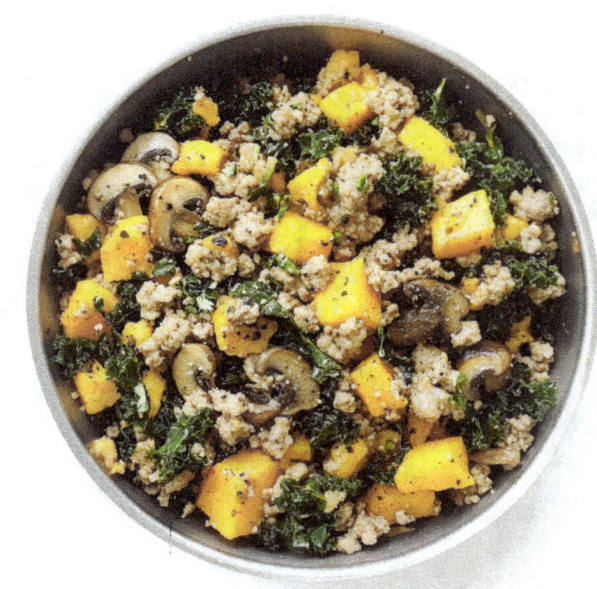

GLUTEN-FREE CREPES

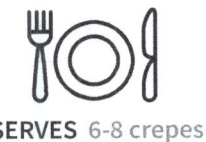 **SERVES** 6-8 crepes

 **PREP** 10 min

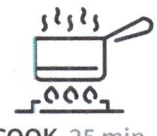 **COOK** 25 min

 **READY IN** 35 min

INGREDIENTS

1 ¼ cups unsweetened almond milk

1 cup gluten-free all-purpose flour

3 tablespoons coconut oil, melted

2 tablespoons maple syrup or honey

2 egg whites

1 ½ teaspoons vanilla extract

¼ teaspoon xanthan gum (optional, omit if your flour blend already contains it)

½ teaspoon salt

DIRECTIONS

1. In a large bowl, whisk the egg whites using a hand mixer or stand mixer until smooth.

2. Gradually add the almond milk, melted coconut oil, maple syrup or honey, vanilla extract, gluten-free flour, xanthan gum (if using), and salt to the egg whites. Mix on medium speed for 1 minute until the batter is completely smooth.

3. Heat a large non-stick (10-12 inch) pan over medium heat and lightly grease it.

4. Pour ¼ cup of the batter into the center of the pan. Lift and tilt the pan to spread the batter into an even circle.

5. Cook the crepe for 30-45 seconds or until the bottom is lightly browned. Carefully flip the crepe and cook for about 30 more seconds until the other side is browned.

6. Remove the crepe from the pan and place it flat on a plate. Continue with the remaining batter.

7. Serve the crepes warm, rolled up or folded into triangles, accompanied by your favorite sweet or savory fillings and toppings.

NOTES

- For thinner crepes, adjust the consistency of the batter by adding a little more almond milk if needed. The batter should be very thin and pourable.

- Cooked crepes can be stored in the refrigerator for up to 5 days or frozen between layers of wax paper in a freezer-safe bag for up to 2 months. Reheat in a warm pan or microwave before serving.

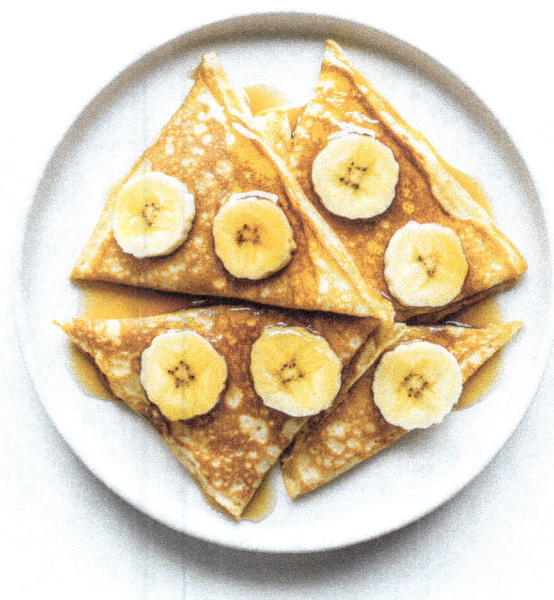

PER SERVING (1 crepe) Calories: 122; Total fat: 5g; Protein: 2g; Carbohydrates: 15g; Fiber: 1g

SWEET POTATO TOAST

SERVES 4-6 slices

PREP 5 min

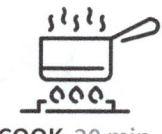
COOK 20 min

READY IN 25 min

INGREDIENTS

1 large sweet potato

1 tablespoon olive oil or coconut oil (optional)

Optional Toppings:

Sweet: sliced banana, almond butter, and maple syrup

Savory: mashed avocado, scrambled egg, and salt

DIRECTIONS

1. Preheat the oven to 400 degrees Fahrenheit and line a large baking sheet with parchment paper.

2. Trim the ends off the sweet potato and slice it lengthwise into ½ inch thick slices. Arrange the slices in a single layer on the baking sheet. If using oil, brush the tops of the sweet potato slices lightly.

3. Bake the sweet potato slices for 20 minutes, or until they are tender when pierced with a fork.

4. Serve the sweet potato toast warm with your preferred toppings or allow them to cool completely and store them in an airtight container in the refrigerator for up to 4-5 days.

5. To reheat, use a toaster or toaster oven set on medium. Alternatively, preheat an oven to 300 degrees Fahrenheit and reheat the slices for 10 minutes.

PER SERVING (1 slice without toppings)
Calories: 55; Total fat: 3g; Protein: 1g;
Carbohydrates: 6g; Fiber: 1g

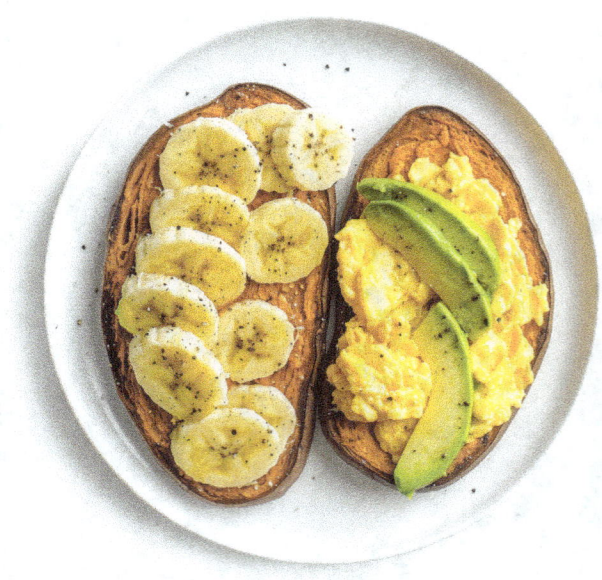

GLUTEN-FREE BAGELS

 **SERVES** 6 bagels

 **PREP** 20 min

 **COOK** 30 min

 **READY IN** 1 h 50 min

INGREDIENTS

1 cup mashed potatoes

2 egg whites

1 cup warm water (105 to 115°F)

3 tablespoons olive oil

2 ¼ cups gluten-free all-purpose flour

1 teaspoon xanthan gum (omit if included in flour)

2 tablespoons psyllium husk powder

1 teaspoon baking powder

2 ¼ teaspoons instant yeast

1 tablespoon maple syrup

¼ teaspoon salt

1 tablespoon sesame seeds (optional, for maintenance phase)

DIRECTIONS

1. Line a baking sheet with parchment. Sift flour, xanthan gum, psyllium husk, baking powder, yeast, and salt in a large bowl.

2. Blend mashed potatoes and egg whites until well combined. Transfer to a mixing bowl; add warm water, maple syrup, and oil. Mix well.

3. Gradually mix dry ingredients into wet to form a sticky dough.

4. Oil hands, form dough into six balls on the baking sheet. Flatten each and poke a hole in the center.

5. Cover and let rise in a warm place for 1 hour.

6. Preheat oven to 350°F. Brush dough with oil and sprinkle with sesame seeds (if using).

7. Bake for 25-30 minutes until golden. Cool on a wire rack.

NOTES

- For the best rise, place the dough in a warm, draft-free area. If your kitchen is cool, an off oven with the light on can create an ideal rising environment.

- After baking, let the bagels cool completely before storing to maintain their texture. They can be stored in an airtight container for up to 5 days in the refrigerator or frozen for up to 2 months.

PER SERVING (1 bagel) Calories: 269; Total fat: 7g; Protein: 4g; Carbohydrates: 43g; Fiber: 3g

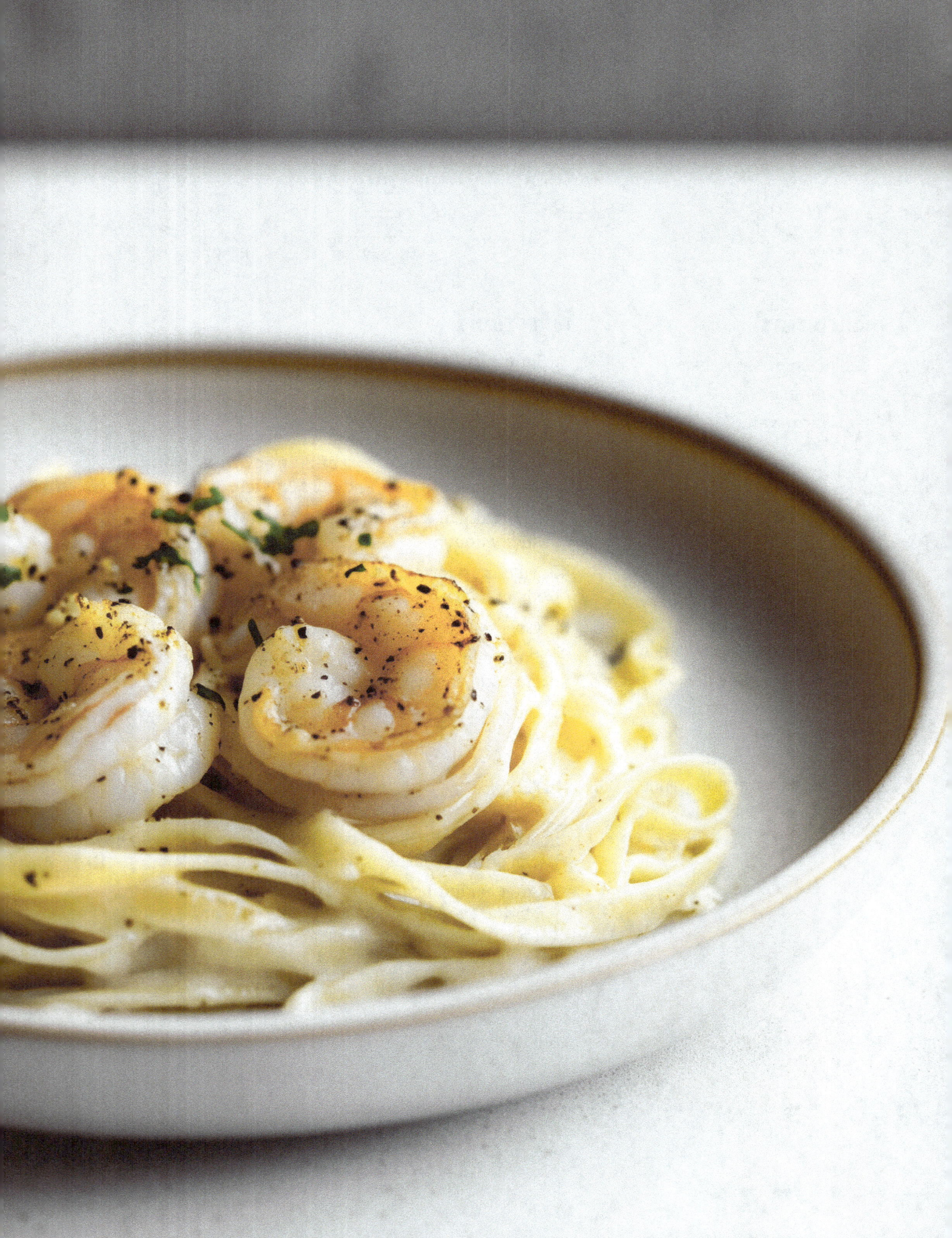

CHAPTER FIVE

MAIN DISHES

SWEET POTATO CHICKEN NUGGETS

  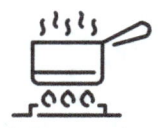 

SERVES 2   **PREP** 15 min   **COOK** 10 min   **READY IN** 25 min

INGREDIENTS

½ pound ground chicken breast (about 1 cup)

1 cup sweet potato, shredded (see note)

1 tablespoon coconut flour

2 teaspoons coconut oil

½ teaspoon salt

DIRECTIONS

1. Preheat the oven to 400 degrees F. Grease a baking sheet with coconut oil or non-stick cooking spray.

2. In a large mixing bowl, combine the ground chicken, shredded sweet potato, coconut oil, coconut flour, and salt. Mix thoroughly until all ingredients are well integrated.

3. Shape the mixture into small, slightly flattened nuggets, about 1-inch in diameter. Arrange the nuggets on the prepared baking sheet.

4. Bake in the preheated oven for 8 to 10 minutes, flipping the nuggets halfway through, until the chicken is fully cooked and the nuggets are golden.

5. Serve the nuggets warm and enjoy!

NOTE

- Use a food processor to shred the sweet potato quickly and efficiently.

PER SERVING (about 6 nuggets)
Calories: 283; Total fat: 8g; Protein: 28g; Carbohydrates: 23g; Fiber: 4g

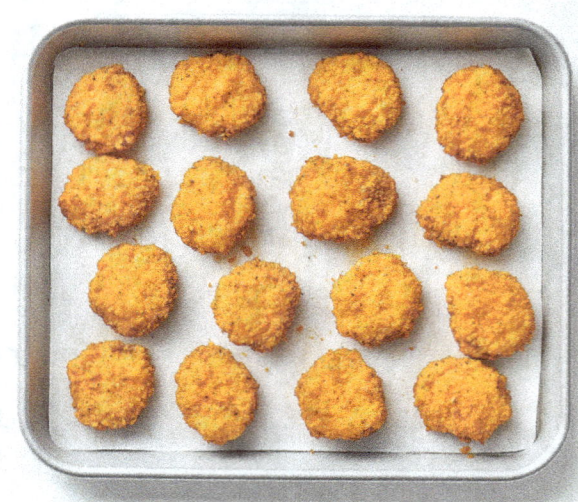

HERB SHRIMP PASTA

SERVES 4

PREP 10 min

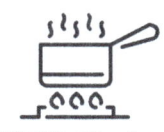

COOK 15 min

READY IN 25 min

INGREDIENTS

1 pound shrimp, peeled and deveined (about 1 ¾ cups)

8 ounces gluten-free pasta (preferably angel hair)

2 teaspoons dried basil

1 teaspoon dried oregano

1 tablespoon olive oil

½ teaspoon salt

¼ cup grated dairy-free Parmesan cheese (optional, for maintenance phase; see p. 175)

DIRECTIONS

1. In a medium saucepan, boil water and cook the pasta according to the package directions.

2. Grease a large skillet with a little olive oil or non-stick cooking spray. Place it over medium-high heat and add the tablespoon of olive oil. Add the oregano, basil, salt, and shrimp to the skillet. Toss to coat the shrimp with the herbs and cook for about 6 to 8 minutes, or until the shrimp are pink and cooked through, turning once.

3. Drain the pasta and toss it with the shrimp mixture in the skillet.

4. Sprinkle with dairy-free Parmesan cheese if using, and serve immediately.

PER SERVING (about 1 cup) Calories: 214; Total fat: 4g; Protein: 31g; Carbohydrates: 10g; Fiber: 2g

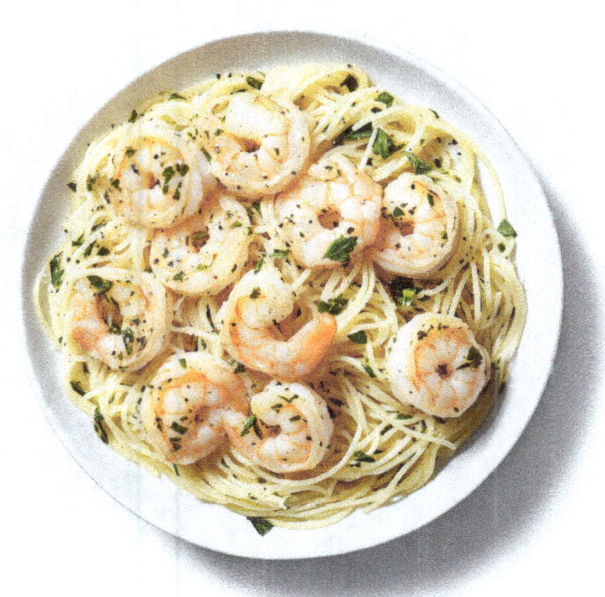

CHICKEN & GREEN BEAN STIR-FRY

SERVES 4

PREP 10 min

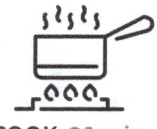

COOK 30 min

READY IN 40 min

INGREDIENTS

1 pound lean ground chicken (about 2 cups)

3 cups green beans, trimmed

⅓ cup chicken broth (optional, see note)

¼ cup coconut aminos

1 tablespoon maple syrup (optional)

2 teaspoons sesame oil

2 teaspoons arrowroot flour (or potato starch)

¼ teaspoon ginger, minced

DIRECTIONS

1. In a small bowl, combine the coconut aminos, chicken broth, and maple syrup (if using). Set aside.

2. Heat a pan over medium heat, add sesame oil and minced ginger, and sauté for 1-2 minutes, stirring frequently.

3. Add the ground chicken and cook for about 5 minutes, or until it's no longer pink.

4. Pour the coconut aminos mixture into the pan, add the green beans, cover, and continue to cook, stirring occasionally, until the green beans are tender, about 15-20 minutes.

5. In a separate small bowl, mix the arrowroot powder with 2 tablespoons of the broth or water until smooth. Add this to the pan, stir well, and cook for an additional minute to thicken the sauce.

6. Remove from heat and serve immediately.

NOTE

- If using store-bought chicken broth, ensure it does not contain potentially irritating ingredients like onion, garlic, or citric acid. Alternatively, consider making your own following the recipe on page 167.

PER SERVING (about 1 cup) Calories: 207; Total fat: 8g; Protein: 7g; Carbohydrates: 10g; Fiber: 2g

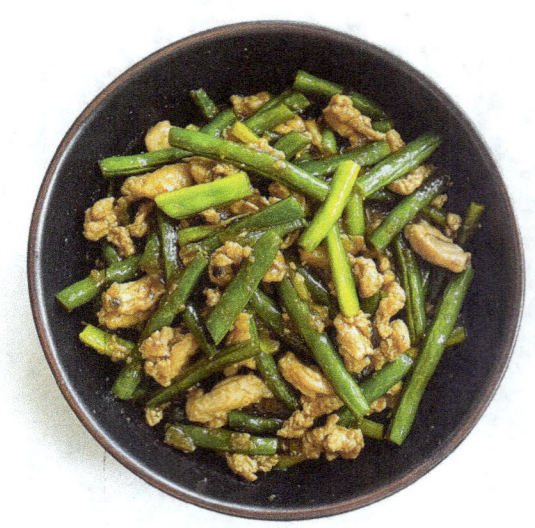

ALMOND CRUSTED CHICKEN

SERVES 2

PREP 15 min

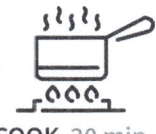
COOK 20 min

READY IN 35 min

INGREDIENTS

1 boneless, skinless chicken breast, cut into strips

½ cup blanched almond flour

1 egg, beaten

½ teaspoon dried oregano

¼ teaspoon dried basil

½ teaspoon salt

Olive oil for drizzling

DIRECTIONS

1. Preheat the oven to 375 degrees F and line a baking sheet with parchment paper.

2. Mix oregano, basil, salt, and almond flour in a small bowl and spread onto a plate or shallow bowl.

3. Place the beaten egg in another shallow bowl.

4. Dredge the chicken in the egg, then in the almond flour mixture, ensuring both sides are well-coated.

5. Place the chicken on the prepared baking sheet and drizzle with olive oil.

6. Bake for 10-15 minutes on one side, flip, and continue baking for another 10 minutes or until golden brown.

7. Serve the chicken warm and enjoy!

NOTE

- Optionally, the chicken breast can be cut into ½-inch thick strips lengthwise before dredging for bite-sized pieces.

PER SERVING (½ of a chicken breast) Calories: 198; Total fat: 9g
Protein: 24g; Carbohydrates: 1g; Fiber: 1g

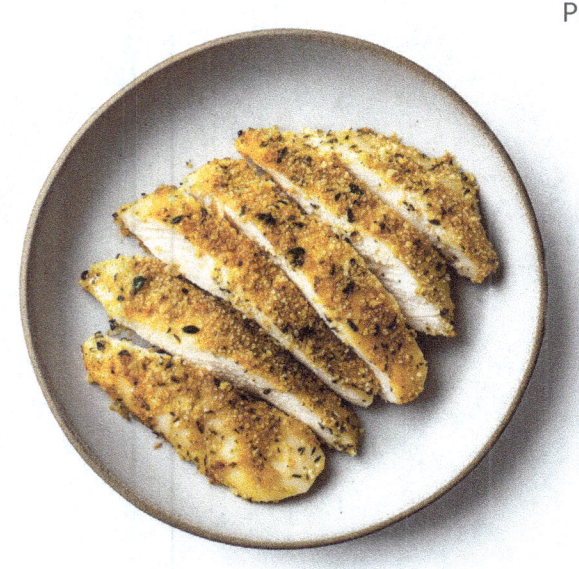

SALMON PATTIES

  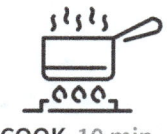 

SERVES 4 patties   **PREP** 15 min   **COOK** 10 min   **READY IN** 25 min

INGREDIENTS

1 can (14.75 oz.) salmon, drained

⅔ cup gluten-free breadcrumbs

1 egg, beaten

1 teaspoon dried dill

½ teaspoon grated lemon zest (optional)

½ teaspoon asafoetida (optional, but recommended)

½ teaspoon salt

2 teaspoons olive oil

DIRECTIONS

1. In a medium bowl, combine the salmon, breadcrumbs, egg, dill, lemon zest, asafoetida, and salt.

2. Use your hands to form the mixture into 4 evenly-sized patties.

3. Heat the olive oil in a large non-stick skillet over medium heat.

4. Place the patties in the skillet and cook until golden brown on each side, about 3-5 minutes per side.

5. Serve the salmon patties with your preferred side dish.

PER SERVING (1 patty) Calories: 230; Total fat: 4g; Protein: 26g; Carbohydrates: 14g; Fiber: 0g

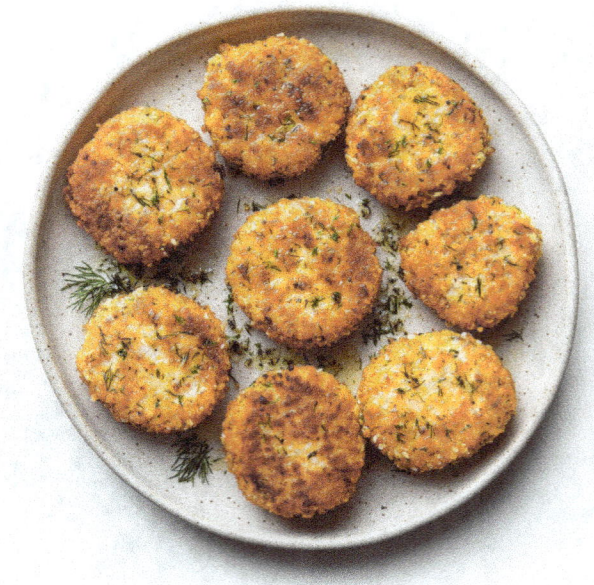

MISO GINGER CHICKEN

SERVES 4

PREP 10 min

COOK 30 min

READY IN 40 min

INGREDIENTS

1 pound chicken breast, cubed (about 2 cups)

½ leek (white part only), diced (optional)

2 ½ tablespoons coconut aminos

1 teaspoon fresh ginger, minced

1 ½ teaspoons white miso paste

2 teaspoons sesame oil

2 teaspoons arrowroot flour (or potato starch)

¼ teaspoon asafoetida (optional)

1 tablespoon olive oil

Sesame seeds (optional, for garnish)

DIRECTIONS

1. Heat the olive oil in a skillet over medium heat. Once hot, add the diced leek and sauté until it begins to soften.

2. Add the cubed chicken to the skillet and cook for 7-10 minutes, flipping occasionally, until the chicken is cooked through.

3. While the chicken cooks, prepare the sauce. In a small bowl, combine the coconut aminos, ginger, miso paste, sesame oil, asafoetida, and arrowroot powder. Whisk well to ensure no clumps remain.

4. Once the chicken is cooked, pour the sauce over it and stir to coat. Continue cooking for an additional 3-5 minutes, until the sauce is heated through and has thickened.

5. Garnish the chicken with sesame seeds (if using). Serve and enjoy!

PER SERVING (about 1 cup) Calories: 257; Total fat: 10g; Protein: 34g; Carbohydrates: 3g; Fiber: 2g

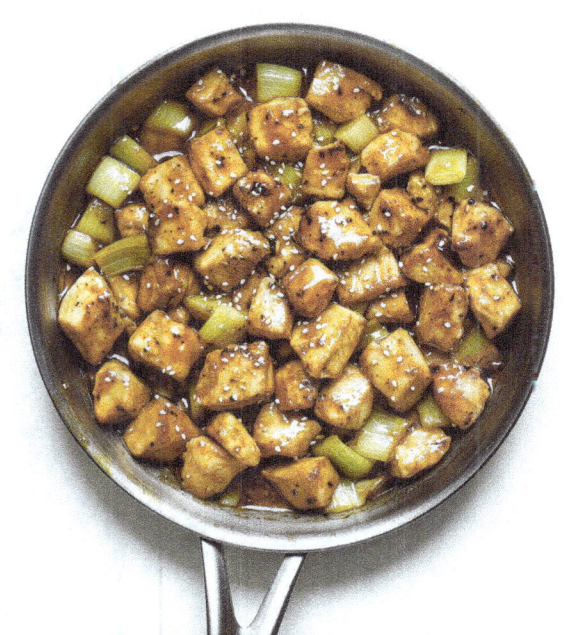

TURKEY STROGANOFF

 **SERVES** 4

 **PREP** 10 min

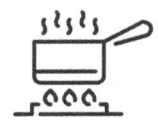 **COOK** 20 min

 **READY IN** 30 min

INGREDIENTS

1 pound lean ground turkey breast (about 2 cups)

8 ounces mushrooms, sliced (about 3 cups)

1 cup unsweetened almond milk

1 ¼ cups chicken broth

1 tablespoon liquid aminos or coconut aminos

2 tablespoons parsley, chopped

1 teaspoon dried thyme

1 teaspoon asafoetida (optional)

2 tablespoons arrowroot flour (or potato starch)

2 teaspoons olive oil, divided

DIRECTIONS

1. In a skillet over medium heat, heat 1 teaspoon of olive oil. Add the ground turkey and cook, stirring occasionally, until it is crumbled and browned, about 5 to 7 minutes. Remove the turkey from the skillet and set aside.

2. In the same skillet, add the remaining teaspoon of olive oil and the sliced mushrooms. Cook for about 3-5 minutes until the mushrooms are tender.

3. In a medium bowl, whisk together the almond milk and arrowroot until smooth, ensuring there are no lumps.

4. Return to the skillet and add the chicken broth, liquid aminos, thyme, asafoetida, and the almond milk mixture to the mushrooms. Bring the mixture to a simmer and let it thicken for about 10 minutes.

5. Add the cooked turkey and parsley to the skillet. Simmer everything together for another 5-8 minutes, allowing the flavors to meld. Season with salt to taste.

6. Serve the turkey stroganoff over cooked rice or pasta for a complete meal.

PER SERVING (about 1 cup)
Calories: 178; Total fat: 4g; Protein: 27g; Carbohydrates: 5g; Fiber: 1g

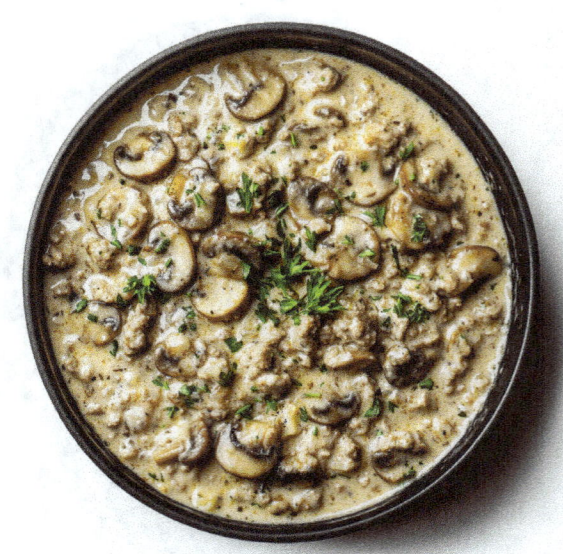

SCALLOPS WITH SPINACH

SERVES 2

PREP 10 min

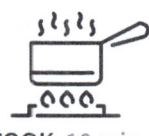

COOK 10 min

READY IN 20 min

INGREDIENTS

12 ounces sea scallops (about 1 ⅓ cups)

3 cups baby spinach

1 tablespoon olive oil

Zest of ½ orange

½ teaspoon salt

DIRECTIONS

1. Heat a large nonstick skillet over medium-high heat and add the olive oil.

2. Season the scallops with ¼ teaspoon of salt and place them in the hot skillet. Cook the scallops for 2 to 3 minutes per side until browned.

3. Transfer the scallops to a platter and cover with aluminum foil to keep warm.

4. In the same skillet, add the spinach, orange zest and the remaining ¼ teaspoon of salt. Cook, stirring frequently, until the spinach wilts, about 3 minutes.

5. Serve the wilted spinach topped with the warm scallops.

NOTE

• Before cooking, remove the small tendon from the side of each scallop using a sharp paring knife for better texture and even cooking.

PER SERVING (½ of the recipe) Calories: 258; Total fat: 8g; Protein: 36g; Carbohydrates: 4g; Fiber: 1g

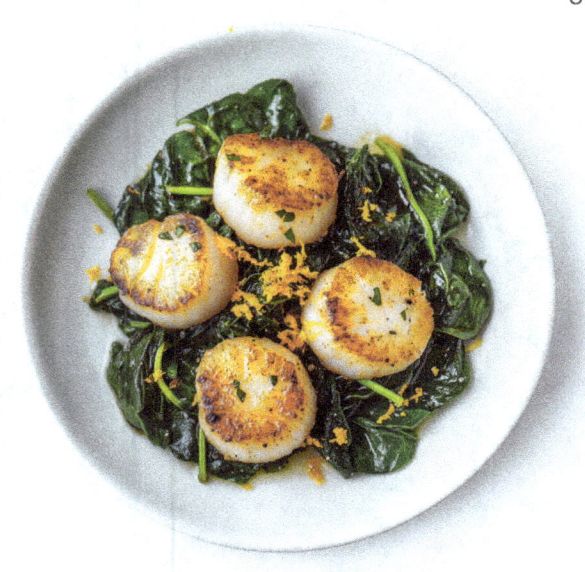

TURKEY & SQUASH RICE CASSEROLE

SERVES 5

PREP 20 min

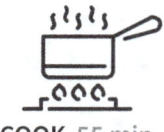
COOK 55 min

READY IN 1 h 15 min

INGREDIENTS

1 pound lean ground turkey (about 2 cups)

1 cup uncooked wild rice

1 ½ pounds butternut squash, peeled and cubed (about 3 ¼ cups)

¼ cup chicken broth or water

2 tablespoons olive oil, divided

2 teaspoons dried oregano

1 teaspoon dried basil

2 tablespoons fresh thyme

½ tablespoon dried rosemary, crushed

⅓ cup dairy-free Parmesan cheese (optional, for maintenance phae, see p. 175)

1 tablespoon salt

DIRECTIONS

1. Cook the wild rice according to package instructions; set aside.

2. Heat 1 tablespoon olive oil in a large skillet or Dutch oven over medium heat. Add ground turkey, half the rosemary, half the thyme, half the oregano, and half the basil. Cook for about 8 minutes until the turkey is thoroughly cooked. Remove from the pan and set aside, retaining the juices.

3. Preheat your oven to 350°F and grease a 9x13 inch casserole dish with olive oil.

4. In the same skillet, add the remaining olive oil, butternut squash, remaining herbs, and broth or water. Cover and cook until the squash is tender, about 8-10 minutes.

5. Combine the cooked squash, rice, turkey with its juices, salt, and half of the Parmesan in the skillet. Mix well, then transfer into the prepared casserole dish.

6. Bake for 15 minutes, sprinkle with the remaining Parmesan, and bake for an additional 5 minutes.

PER SERVING (about 1 cup)
Calories: 349; Total fat: 8g; Protein: 34g; Carbohydrates: 31g; Fiber: 6g

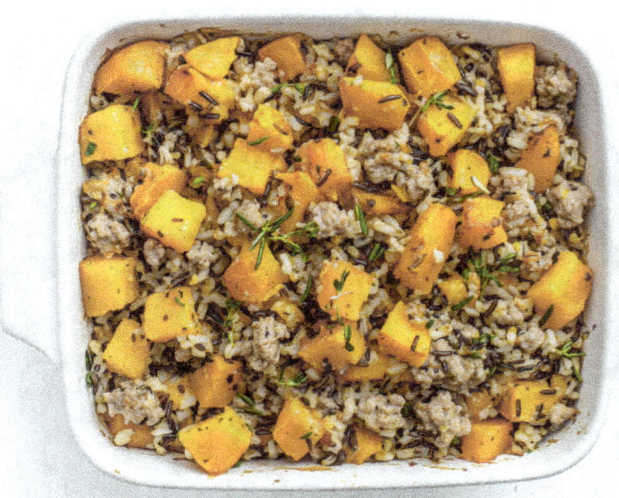

BROILED CHICKEN KABOBS

SERVES 2

PREP 20 min

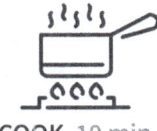

COOK 10 min

READY IN 30 min

INGREDIENTS

1 boneless, skinless chicken breast, cut into 1-inch pieces

1 cup zucchini, cut into 1-inch pieces

1 cup whole button mushrooms, stems removed

1 teaspoon olive oil

½ teaspoon dried oregano

½ teaspoon dried basil

¼ teaspoon dried rosemary

¼ teaspoon fresh parsley

¼ teaspoon salt

DIRECTIONS

1. In a medium bowl, mix together oregano, basil, rosemary, parsley, salt, and olive oil.

2. Add chicken pieces to the bowl and toss to coat evenly. Let marinate for 5 minutes.

3. Preheat the broiler for 15 to 20 minutes.

4. Mix mushrooms and zucchini into the bowl with the chicken.

5. Thread chicken, zucchini, and mushrooms alternately onto skewers.

6. Line a baking sheet with foil or spray with non-stick cooking spray. Arrange kabobs in a single layer.

7. Broil kabobs for about 5 minutes on each side, turning once, until chicken is cooked through.

8. Serve with your choice of side dish.

PER SERVING (½ of the recipe) Calories: 145; Total fat: 5g; Protein: 20g; Carbohydrates: 2g; Fiber: 1g

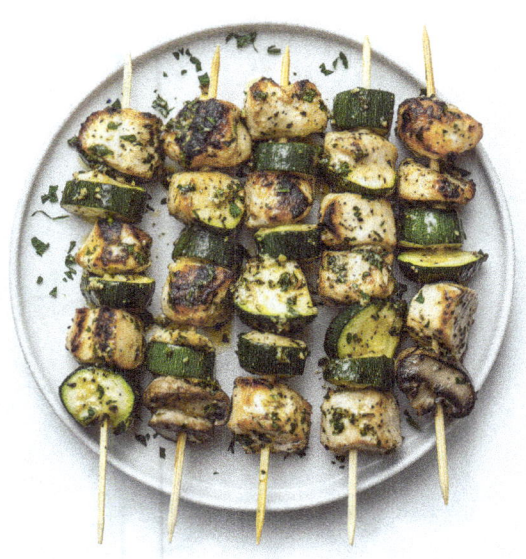

CRAB CAKES

SERVES 2

PREP 30 min

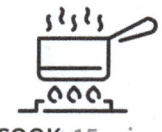
COOK 15 min

READY IN 45 min

INGREDIENTS

8 ounces lump crab meat, drained

⅔ cup gluten-free breadcrumbs

1 large egg, beaten

2 tablespoons fresh cilantro, chopped

1 teaspoon lime zest

¼ teaspoon salt

DIRECTIONS

1. Preheat the oven to 450 degrees F and lightly grease a rimmed baking sheet with olive oil or non-stick cooking spray.

2. In a medium bowl, mix together the crab meat, beaten egg, breadcrumbs, cilantro, lime zest, and salt. Cover and chill in the refrigerator for 25 minutes.

3. Shape the crab mixture into two or three patties and place them on the prepared baking sheet.

4. Bake for 15 minutes or until the crab cakes are golden brown.

5. Serve warm with your preferred side dish.

PER SERVING (½ of the recipe)
Calories: 261; Total fat: 3g; Protein: 25g; Carbohydrates: 29g; Fiber: 0g

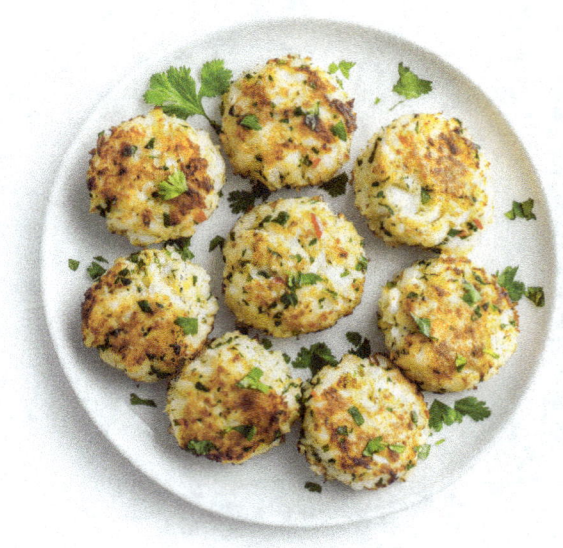

CRISPY SESAME TEMPEH

SERVES 2

PREP 15 min

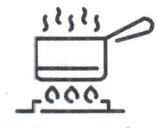

COOK 15 min

READY IN 30 min

INGREDIENTS

8 ounces tempeh, cut into ¾-inch cubes (about 1 ⅓ cups)

1 tablespoon coconut aminos

½ teaspoon salt

1 tablespoon olive oil

Stir-fry Sauce:

2 tablespoons coconut aminos

2 tablespoons water

1 tablespoon maple syrup

1 teaspoon sesame oil

1 teaspoon ginger, finely minced (optional)

1 tablespoon sesame seeds (optional, for garnish)

DIRECTIONS

1. In a medium pot, cover the tempeh cubes with just enough water to reach the top. Add 1 tablespoon of coconut aminos and ½ teaspoon of salt. Bring to a boil, then cover, reduce the heat to medium-low, and simmer for 10 minutes.

2. While the tempeh simmers, whisk together all sauce ingredients in a small bowl and set it aside near the stove.

3. Once the tempeh is done simmering, drain and pat it dry with paper towels to remove excess moisture.

4. Heat olive oil in a large skillet over medium heat. Lightly season the oil with salt. Add the tempeh and sauté until each side is deeply golden, about 5 minutes per side.

5. Pour the prepared stir-fry sauce over the tempeh, reduce the heat slightly, and allow the sauce to reduce by half, frequently spooning it over the tempeh until it thickens.

6. Serve the crispy tempeh over a bed of rice, accompanied by steamed broccoli and other vegetables if desired. Garnish with sesame seeds and drizzle with any additional sauce.

PER SERVING (½ of the recipe) Calories: 305; Total fat: 16g; Protein: 23g; Carbohydrates: 16g; Fiber: 4g

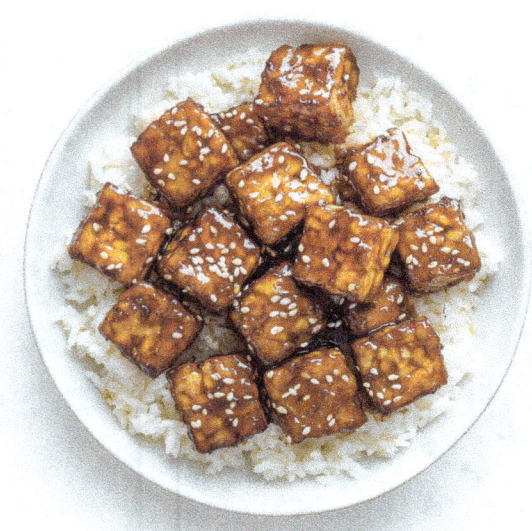

SWEET POTATO NOODLES SKILLET

SERVES 4

PREP 15 min

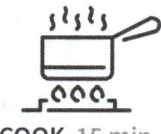
COOK 15 min

READY IN 30 min

INGREDIENTS

1 pound ground turkey breast (about 2 cups)

1 medium sweet potato, spiralized

1 cup baby spinach

1 tablespoon olive oil

½ teaspoon dried oregano

½ teaspoon ground cumin

Salt to taste

DIRECTIONS

1. Heat the olive oil in a skillet over medium heat.

2. Add the ground turkey to the skillet, seasoning it with salt, oregano, and cumin. Cook until it's halfway done.

3. Introduce the spiralized sweet potato noodles to the skillet. Cook for about 5 to 8 minutes, tossing occasionally with a spatula. Add a few tablespoons of water if needed to prevent the noodles from sticking.

4. Stir in the baby spinach and cook for an additional 2 minutes, or until the spinach has wilted.

5. Serve the skillet warm.

NOTE

- Sweet potato noodles can be made using a spiralizer, or pre-made noodles can be purchased from a supermarket for convenience.

PER SERVING (about ¾ cup)
Calories: 175; Total fat: 4g; Protein: 26g; Carbohydrates: 4g; Fiber: 1g

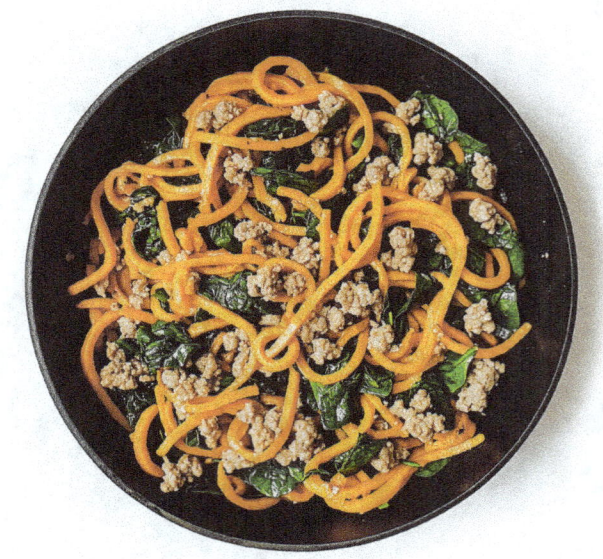

PUMPKIN PASTA

 SERVES 4

 PREP 10 min

 COOK 20 min

 READY IN 30 min

INGREDIENTS

16 ounces gluten-free penne pasta or other pasta of choice

1 cup canned pumpkin puree

½ leek (white part only), diced

1 tablespoon arrowroot flour (or potato starch)

2 tablespoons coconut cream (optional)

2 cups unsweetened almond milk

2 teaspoons fresh chopped sage

2 teaspoons fresh chopped thyme

2 tablespoons olive oil

¼ cup nutritional yeast

⅛ teaspoon nutmeg (optional, for maintenance phase)

1-1 ½ teaspoons salt

DIRECTIONS

1. Cook the pasta in a large pot of boiling water according to package instructions.

2. In a pan, sauté the diced leek in olive oil over low heat until it starts to soften.

3. Add the sage and thyme to the pan and cook for about 5 minutes, allowing the flavors to blend.

4. Transfer the sautéed leek and herbs to a blender or food processor. Add the pumpkin puree, almond milk, coconut cream, nutritional yeast, nutmeg, and salt. Process until smooth.

5. Add the arrowroot starch to the mixture in the blender and pulse a few times to incorporate. The sauce will be thin at this stage.

6. Pour the sauce into a large pan and heat over low heat. Simmer for about 5 minutes, or until the sauce thickens.

7. Taste and adjust the seasoning if needed.

8. Combine the thickened sauce with the cooked pasta, tossing to coat evenly.

9. Serve immediately and enjoy!

PER SERVING (about 1 ½ cups) Calories: 291; Total fat: 10g; Protein: 7g; Carbohydrates: 41g; Fiber: 4g

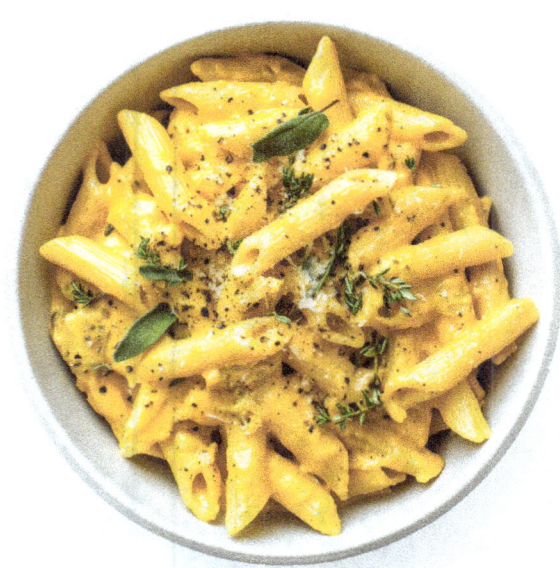

BUTTERNUT SQUASH RISOTTO

SERVES 4

PREP 10 min

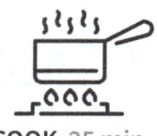
COOK 25 min

READY IN 35 min

INGREDIENTS

2 tablespoons olive oil

1 cup leek (white part only), diced

8 sage leaves, chopped

1 cup Arborio rice or short-grain rice

2 heaping cups of butternut squash, cubed (buying pre-cut squash can save prep time)

2 cups vegetable or chicken broth (or water)

2–3 handfuls baby spinach or chopped kale

½ teaspoon salt, more to taste

½ teaspoon nutmeg (optional, but recommended)

DIRECTIONS

1. Thoroughly rinse the leeks after slicing to remove any dirt and help them soften faster.

2. Heat olive oil in a large skillet over medium heat. Add the leeks and sauté for about 2 minutes until they begin to soften.

3. Add the chopped sage and Arborio rice to the skillet. Stir continuously for another 2 minutes until the rice is well-coated and slightly toasted.

4. Mix in the cubed butternut squash and cook for a few minutes, allowing some browning on the bottom of the skillet.

5. Gradually add the broth, stirring constantly. Bring the mixture to a simmer, then reduce the heat to low. Continue cooking, stirring frequently, until the rice and squash are tender and the risotto is creamy, about 18-20 minutes. Add more broth if needed to reach desired consistency.

6. Stir in the spinach or kale until wilted and incorporated into the risotto. Season with salt and optionally, nutmeg. Adjust the seasoning to your taste.

7. Serve the risotto warm and enjoy!

PER SERVING (about 1 ½ cups)
Calories: 277; Total fat: 7g; Protein: 4g;
Carbohydrates: 46g; Fiber: 4g

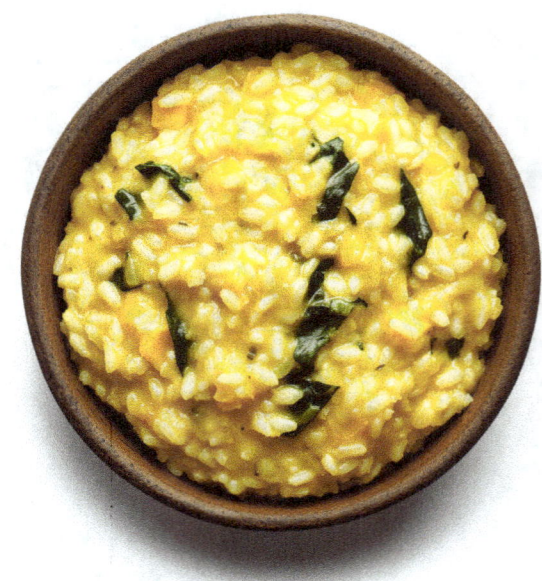

MAPLE ROSEMARY GRILLED CHICKEN

SERVES 2

PREP 10 min

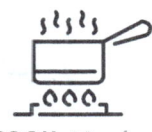
COOK 10 min

READY IN 50 min

INGREDIENTS

1 boneless, skinless chicken breast

1 tablespoon maple syrup

1 tablespoon coconut aminos

1 ½ tablespoons olive oil (divided)

¼ cup diced leek (white part only)

1 tablespoon fresh rosemary, chopped

2 teaspoons grated lemon zest

Salt to taste

Fresh rosemary sprigs (optional, for garnish)

DIRECTIONS

1. In a small bowl, combine the maple syrup, coconut aminos, 1 tablespoon olive oil, diced leek, chopped rosemary, lemon zest, and salt. Mix well.

2. Place the chicken breasts in a large Ziploc bag and pour in the marinade. Ensure the chicken is thoroughly coated. Seal the bag and refrigerate to marinate for at least 30 minutes, or overnight, turning occasionally.

3. Heat a grill or grill skillet over medium-high heat.

4. Remove the chicken from the marinade, discarding the leftover marinade. Brush the chicken with the remaining ½ tablespoon of olive oil and season again with a little more salt. Grill the chicken, turning occasionally, until it is fully cooked and the internal temperature reaches 165°F (about 10 minutes).

5. Place the grilled chicken on a plate and garnish with fresh rosemary sprigs, if desired.

PER SERVING (½ of a chicken breast) Calories: 190; Total fat: 7g; Protein: 18g; Carbohydrates: 10g; Fiber: 0g

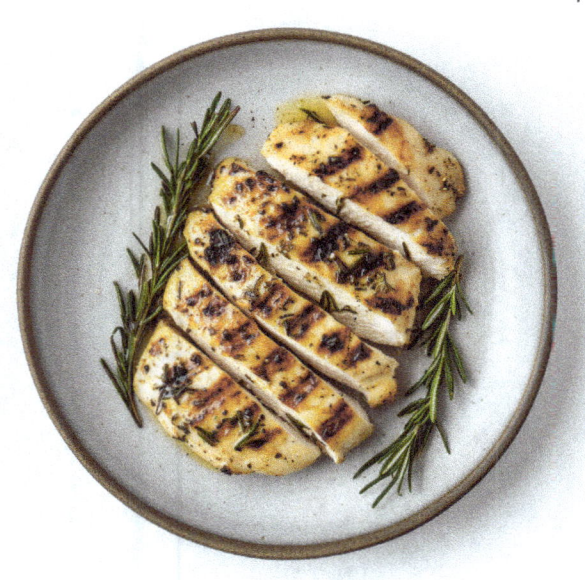

AIRFRYER CHICKEN TENDERS

SERVES 2

PREP 10 min

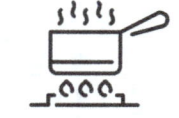
COOK 15-20 min

READY IN 25-30 min

INGREDIENTS

1 skinless chicken breast

⅓ cup gluten-free all-purpose flour

1 egg, beaten

1 tablespoon oregano

1 tablespoon parsley flakes

1 teaspoon salt

Olive oil cooking spray (optional)

DIRECTIONS

1. Start by slicing the chicken breast into long, 1-inch wide strips to make tenders. Ensure each piece is of even thickness for uniform cooking.

2. Set the air fryer to 390 degrees Fahrenheit to preheat.

3. In a shallow dish, mix the flour, oregano, parsley flakes, and salt. In another shallow dish, place the beaten egg.

4. Dip each tender first into the flour mixture, ensuring it's completely coated. Shake off any excess flour. Then dip it into the beaten egg, followed by another coat in the flour mixture. Shake off excess flour again.

5. If desired, lightly spray the chicken with cooking spray to enhance crispiness. Arrange the chicken tenders in a single layer in the air fryer basket, ensuring they do not overlap.

6. Cook the chicken tenders for 15-20 minutes, or until they are golden brown and reach an internal temperature of 165 degrees Fahrenheit. Turn the tenders halfway through cooking to ensure even browning.

7. Remove the chicken tenders from the air fryer and serve warm with your favorite dipping sauces.

PER SERVING (½ of the recipe)
Calories: 209; Total fat: 5g; Protein: 22g; Carbohydrates: 15g; Fiber: 0g

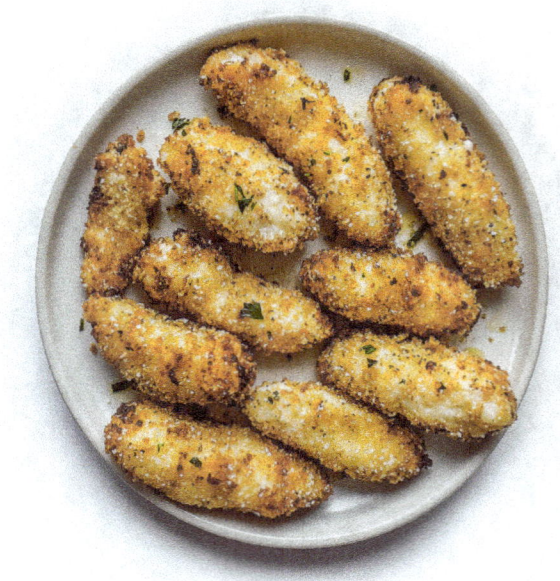

LENTIL MEATBALLS

SERVES 4

PREP 20 min

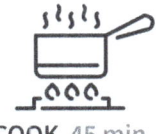
COOK 45 min

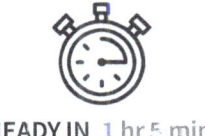
READY IN 1 hr 5 min

INGREDIENTS

1 cup uncooked lentils (black, green, or brown)

½ cup uncooked quinoa

1 tablespoon olive oil

1 teaspoon fennel seeds

½ teaspoon asafoetida (optional)

⅓ cup fresh cilantro, chopped

6 ounces firm tofu, pressed and patted dry

1 teaspoon salt

DIRECTIONS

1. Bring 3 cups of water to a boil in a small pot, add lentils and fennel seeds. Cover, reduce heat to low, and simmer for 25 minutes. Drain and let cool.

2. In another pot, bring 1 cup of water to a boil, add quinoa, cover, reduce heat to low and simmer for 15 minutes. Turn off the heat but leave covered to steam.

3. Preheat the oven to 400°F (200°C) and line a baking sheet with parchment paper.

4. In a food processor, pulse half of the cooked lentils with the cooked quinoa until resembling coarse sand, and transfer to a large mixing bowl.

5. Add remaining lentils, cilantro, salt, and asafoetida to the bowl and mix.

6. Blend the tofu and olive oil in the food processor until smooth, then mix into the lentil mixture.

7. Knead the mixture briefly, then with wet hands, form into ping-pong-sized balls and place on the prepared baking sheet.

8. Bake for 20-25 minutes, or until the meatballs are firm and slightly golden.

9. Serve warm with your favorite sauce or as part of a meal.

PER SERVING (4 meatballs) Calories: 209; Total fat: 7g; Protein: 12g; Carbohydrates: 20g; Fiber: 5g

MUSHROOM & SPINACH GNOCCHI

 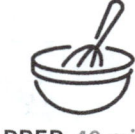 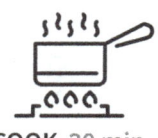 

SERVES 4   **PREP** 40 min   **COOK** 30 min   **READY IN** 1 hr 10 min

INGREDIENTS

1 pound potatoes, washed (about 1⅔ cups)

1 cup gluten-free all-purpose flour

1 large egg

3 cups spinach

8 ounces white mushrooms (about 2 ⅓ cups)

½ leek (white part only), diced (or ½ teaspoon asafoetida)

1 tablespoon dried basil

½ teaspoon fresh thyme

1 tablespoon olive oil

½ teaspoon salt, plus more to taste

DIRECTIONS

1. In a large pot, boil the potatoes until tender. Remove, let cool slightly, then peel and pass through a potato ricer.

2. On a flat surface, mix the flour and salt. Make a well in the center, add the riced potatoes and the egg. Mix with your fingers to form a soft dough. It should not stick to your fingers.

3. On a lightly floured surface, roll small portions of dough into ropes and cut into ¾ inch pieces. Press each piece against the tines of a fork to form ridges. Lightly flour the shaped gnocchi to prevent sticking. Let rest for 20 minutes.

4. Rinse and trim the spinach and mushrooms. Slice the mushrooms.

5. In a large skillet over medium heat, add olive oil. Once hot, add mushrooms, diced leek (or asafoetida), dried basil, and thyme. Cook until the mushrooms are tender and leeks are translucent, about 5-7 minutes.

6. Mix in the spinach and cook until wilted, about 3-5 minutes.

7. Turn off the heat, add the gnocchi directly to the skillet, and toss with the vegetables. Season with additional salt to taste.

PER SERVING (about 1 cup)
Calories: 265; Total fat: 5g; Protein: 7g; Carbohydrates: 42g; Fiber: 4g

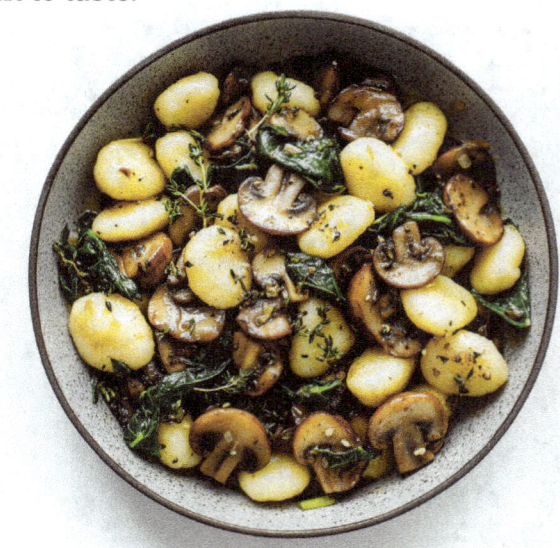

CREAMY BROCCOLI POTATO SOUP

SERVES 2

PREP 20 min

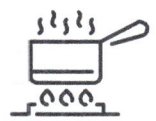

COOK 20 min

READY IN 40 min

INGREDIENTS

3 cups broccoli, chopped

4 medium potatoes, peeled and cubed

1 cup carrots, shredded

2 cups vegetable broth (or water)

⅓ cup canned coconut milk

2 tablespoons arrowroot flour (or potato starch)

¼ cup nutritional yeast

¼ teaspoon salt, plus more to taste

DIRECTIONS

1. In a medium stockpot, bring the vegetable broth (or water) to a boil. Add the potatoes, broccoli, carrots, and salt. Cook for about 15 minutes, or until the vegetables are tender.

2. While the vegetables are cooking, in a small bowl whisk together the arrowroot flour, coconut milk, and ¼ cup water until smooth. You can also blend this mixture for a smoother consistency.

3. Once the vegetables are tender, reduce the heat to a simmer and slowly stir in the coconut milk mixture. Continue to cook for another minute, allowing the soup to thicken.

4. Stir in the nutritional yeast. Taste and adjust seasoning with additional salt if needed.

5. Remove the soup from heat and serve warm.

PER SERVING (½ of the recipe) Calories: 445; Total fat: 7g; Protein: 17g; Carbohydrates: 63g; Fiber: 17g

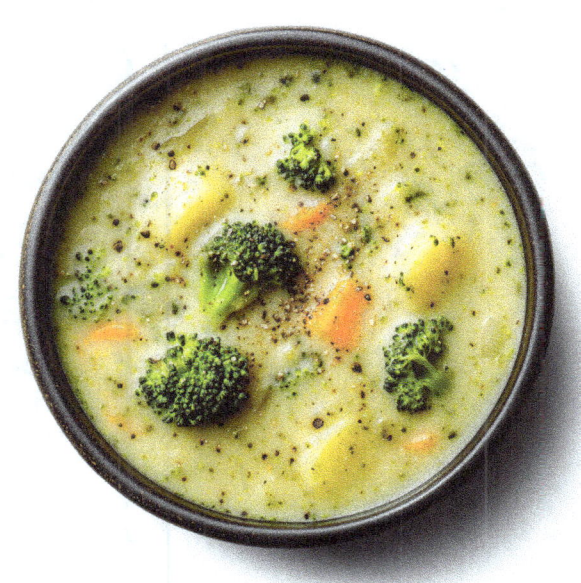

PECAN CRUSTED SALMON

SERVES 2

PREP 15 min

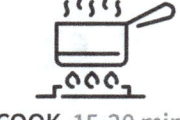
COOK 15-20 min

READY IN 30-35 min

INGREDIENTS

2 (4 oz.) salmon fillets

¼ cup pecans, finely chopped

1 tablespoon maple syrup

1 tablespoon olive oil

1 tablespoon fresh parsley, chopped

¼ teaspoon paprika (optional, if tolerated)

¼ teaspoon salt, plus more for seasoning

DIRECTIONS

1. Set your oven to 425°F.

2. In a small bowl, mix together the chopped pecans, maple syrup, paprika, olive oil, chopped parsley, and salt to create the crust mixture.

3. Lightly season the salmon fillets with a little more salt (if desired) and place them on a greased baking sheet.

4. Spoon the pecan mixture evenly onto the top of each salmon fillet.

5. Place in the oven and bake for 15-20 minutes. The exact time will depend on the thickness of the fillets. Check the salmon after 15 minutes; it should reach an internal temperature of 145°F at the thickest part without overcooking.

6. Remove the salmon from the oven and serve immediately with your choice of side dishes.

PER SERVING (1 salmon fillet)
Calories: 324; Total fat: 19g; Protein: 29g; Carbohydrates: 6g; Fiber: 0g

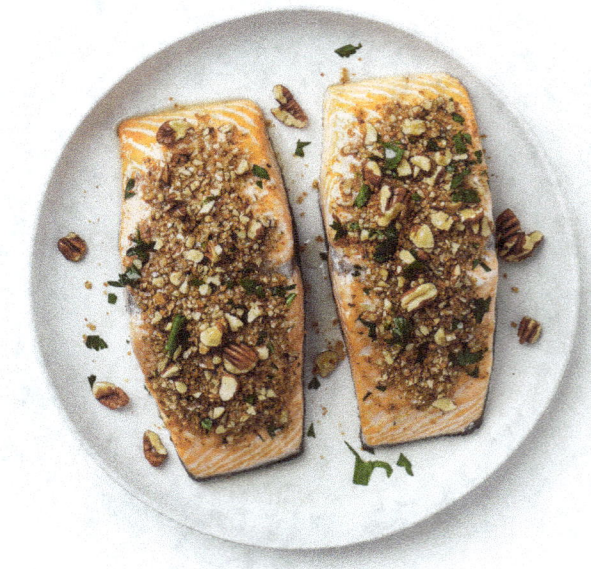

STUFFED CABBAGE ROLLS

SERVES 4

PREP 20 min

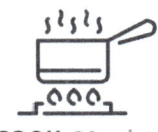

COOK 30 min

READY IN 50 min

INGREDIENTS

1 pound lean ground turkey (about 2 cups)

8 cabbage leaves

⅔ cup water

⅓ cup uncooked white rice

1 ½ cups diced vegetables (such as carrots and celery)

1 egg, beaten

2 teaspoons sesame oil, divided

1 teaspoon grated ginger

3 tablespoons coconut aminos, divided

1 tablespoon olive oil

¼ teaspoon asafoetida (optional)

¼ cup chicken broth or water

DIRECTIONS

1. In a saucepan, bring water and rice to a boil. Reduce heat to low, cover, and simmer until the rice is tender and the liquid has been absorbed, about 20 minutes.

2. Meanwhile, bring a separate pot of lightly salted water to a boil. Blanch the cabbage leaves a few at a time for about a minute until slightly tender. Remove with tongs and set aside to cool.

3. In a skillet over medium heat, heat the olive oil. Add the diced vegetables and ginger, cooking until they start to soften, about 5 minutes. Remove from heat and let cool.

4. In a large bowl, combine the cooked rice, cooled vegetables, ground turkey, and egg. Stir in 2 tablespoons coconut aminos, asafoetida, and 1 teaspoon sesame oil until well mixed.

5. Set your oven to 400 degrees Fahrenheit.

6. Lay a blanched cabbage leaf flat with the stem facing you. Spoon about ¼ cup of the mixture onto the base of each leaf. Roll up the leaf, securing the filling inside. Repeat with all cabbage leaves.

7. In a small bowl, whisk together the remaining coconut aminos, sesame oil, and chicken broth.

8. If there is any leftover mixture, cook it in a skillet over medium heat until the meat is thoroughly cooked, about 7-10 minutes.

9. Place the cabbage rolls in a baking dish and pour the sauce mixture over them. Bake for 30 minutes, or until the cabbage is browned on top and the internal temperature reaches 160 degrees Fahrenheit.

10. Remove from oven and serve.

PER SERVING (2 stuffed cabbage rolls) Calories: 323; Total fat: 9g; Protein: 38g; Carbohydrates: 18g; Fiber: 2g

BUTTERNUT SQUASH SOUP

SERVES 2

PREP 10 min

COOK 40 min

READY IN 50 min

INGREDIENTS

1 butternut squash, peeled and cubed

2 medium carrots, chopped

2 celery stalks, roughly chopped

½ leek (white part only), washed and sliced

3 ½ cups vegetable broth or water

½ cup unsweetened coconut milk (or other plant-based milk)

2 teaspoons olive oil

¾ teaspoon sage

½ teaspoon salt

DIRECTIONS

1. In a large pot, heat the olive oil over medium heat. Add the leek, carrots, and celery. Sauté until they begin to soften, about 5 minutes.

2. Add the cubed butternut squash to the pot, stir in the sage and salt. Cook for another 2-3 minutes.

3. Pour in the vegetable broth or water. Bring to a boil, then reduce the heat to low and let it simmer for about 20-25 minutes, or until all vegetables are tender.

4. Using an immersion blender, blend the soup directly in the pot until it is smooth. Alternatively, carefully transfer the soup to a blender in batches and blend until smooth.

5. Stir in the coconut milk and heat the soup for an additional 5 minutes on low heat. Adjust seasoning as needed.

6. Serve the soup warm, optionally garnished with a swirl of coconut milk or fresh herbs.

PER SERVING (½ of the recipe)
Calories: 293; Total fat: 7g; Protein: 5.5g;
Carbohydrates: 42g; Fiber: 17g

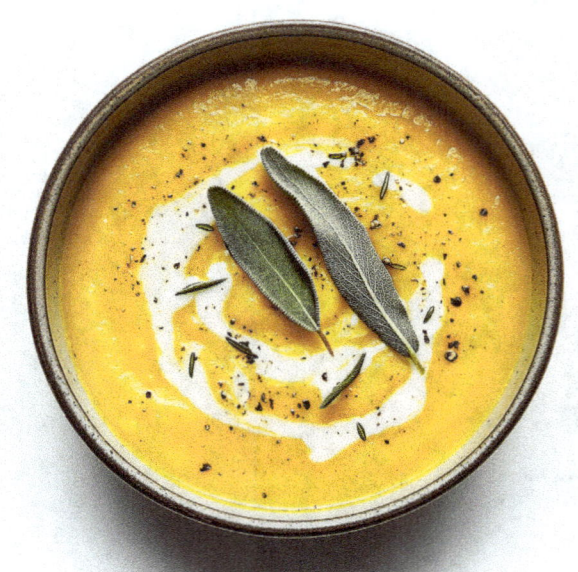

MISO SOUP

 **SERVES** 2

 **PREP** 20 min

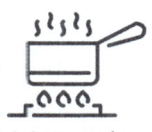 **COOK** 5 min

 **READY IN** 25 min

INGREDIENTS

3 cups vegetable broth

¼ cup dried wakame

2 tablespoons white miso paste

6 ounces tofu (soft or firm), cut into ½-inch cubes

¼ cup leek, thinly sliced

DIRECTIONS

1. In a bowl, cover the wakame with warm water by 1 inch and let sit for about 15 minutes, or until fully reconstituted. Drain in a strainer.

2. In a small bowl, mix the miso paste with ½ cup of the vegetable broth, stirring until smooth. This will help prevent clumps of miso in the soup.

3. In a medium saucepan, bring the remaining vegetable broth to a simmer over medium-high heat.

4. Add the tofu and rehydrated wakame to the broth. Let it simmer for 1 minute, then remove from heat to prevent the tofu from breaking down.

5. Gently stir in the miso mixture and sliced leek into the hot broth. Serve the soup warm, ensuring it's thoroughly mixed.

PER SERVING (about 1 ½ cups) Calories: 133; Total fat: 5g; Protein: 12g; Carbohydrates: 7g; Fiber: 2g

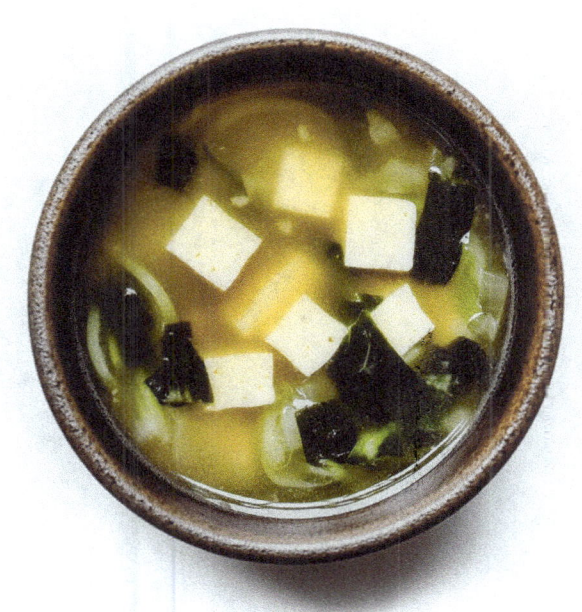

CREAMY MACARONI PASTA

SERVES 4

PREP 10 min

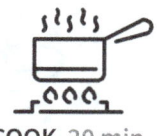
COOK 20 min

READY IN 30 min

INGREDIENTS

8 ounces gluten-free macaroni pasta

2 ½ cups cauliflower, chopped

½ cup water

¼-½ teaspoon asafoetida

¼ cup nutritional yeast

1 teaspoon grated lemon zest

1-2 tablespoons coconut aminos

¼ teaspoon turmeric

Salt to taste

DIRECTIONS

1. Prepare the gluten-free macaroni pasta according to the package instructions. Drain and set aside.

2. While the pasta cooks, steam or boil the cauliflower in a pot of water until tender, about 10-15 minutes.

3. In a blender, combine the cooked cauliflower, water, asafoetida, nutritional yeast, lemon zest, coconut aminos, turmeric, and salt. Blend until smooth, adding more water as needed to reach a creamy consistency.

4. Return the pasta to a large pot or skillet over low heat, then pour in the sauce. Stir until the pasta is fully coated and the sauce is warmed through. Adjust salt if needed.

5. Serve warm and enjoy!

PER SERVING (about 1 cup)
Calories: 238; Total fat: 1g; Protein: 8g;
Carbohydrates: 45g; Fiber: 4g

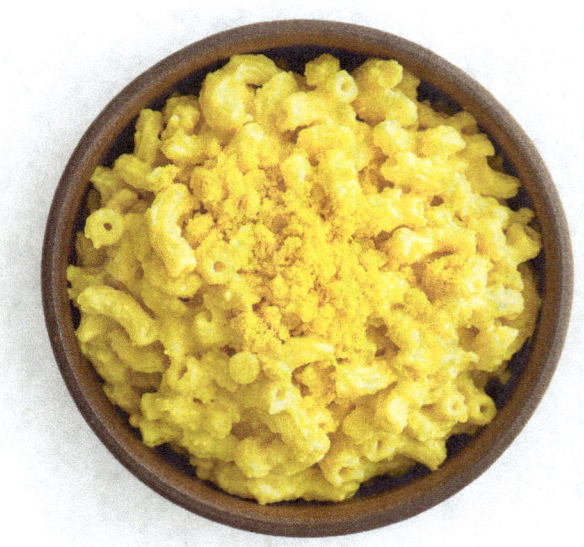

THAI COCONUT SOUP

 **SERVES** 4

 **PREP** 30 min

 **COOK** 30 min

 **READY IN** 1 hour

INGREDIENTS

1 skinless chicken breast, cut into bite-size pieces

2 medium carrots, cut into matchsticks

½ cup mushrooms, sliced

1 celeriac root, diced (optional)

1 cup kale, de-stemmed and cut into 1-inch pieces

½ leek (white part only), diced

1 tablespoon coconut oil

1-2 teaspoons turmeric

½ teaspoon cumin

1 teaspoon fresh ginger, grated

¼ teaspoon asafoetida (optional)

1 (14 oz.) can lite coconut milk

3-4 cups vegetable broth

½ teaspoon salt (or to taste)

DIRECTIONS

1. In a large pot or Dutch oven, heat the coconut oil over medium heat. Add the diced leek and grated ginger, sautéing until the leek is soft.

2. Stir in turmeric, cumin, and asafoetida (if using), cooking for another 2 minutes to release the flavors.

3. Pour in the vegetable broth and coconut milk, then add the mushrooms, carrots, and celeriac root (if using). Bring the mixture to a simmer and cook for about 12-15 minutes until the vegetables begin to soften.

4. Add the chicken pieces to the soup, allowing them to cook and infuse the broth for about 10 minutes, or until fully cooked.

5. Stir in the kale and cook for an additional 2 minutes until it's slightly wilted.

6. Season the soup with salt, adjusting according to your taste preferences.

7. Serve warm and enjoy!

PER SERVING (about 1 ½ cups) Calories: 187; Total fat: 10g; Protein: 11g; Carbohydrates: 9g; Fiber: 2g

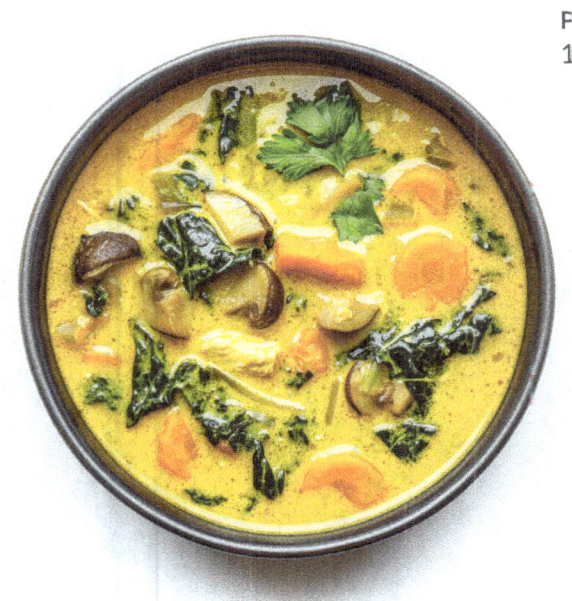

BAKED FALAFEL

 **SERVES** 4

 **PREP** 15 min

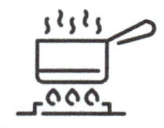 **COOK** 30 min

 **READY IN** 45 min

INGREDIENTS

1 cup dried chickpeas, soaked (see note)

½ teaspoon ground cumin

½ teaspoon asafoetida (optional)

½ cup fresh cilantro, chopped

½ cup fresh parsley, chopped

1 teaspoon salt

2 tablespoons + 1 teaspoon olive oil

DIRECTIONS

1. Set your oven rack in the middle position and preheat to 375 degrees Fahrenheit. Coat a large rimmed baking sheet evenly with 2 tablespoons of olive oil.

2. In a food processor, blend the soaked and drained chickpeas, parsley, cilantro, asafoetida (if using), cumin, salt, and 1 teaspoon of olive oil until smooth, about 1 minute.

3. Scoop about 2 tablespoons of the mixture at a time and shape into small patties, each about 2 inches wide and ½ inch thick. Place each patty on the oiled baking sheet.

4. Bake for 25 to 30 minutes, turning the falafels halfway through, until they are deeply golden on both sides.

5. Store leftovers in the refrigerator for up to 4 days or freeze for several months for prolonged freshness.

NOTE

- Ensure chickpeas are well-soaked, ideally overnight, for best results. Do not substitute with canned chickpeas as they are too moist and will not hold the falafel patties together effectively.

PER SERVING (about 3 falafel balls)
Calories: 189; Total fat: 9g; Protein: 7g;
Carbohydrates: 16g; Fiber: 5g

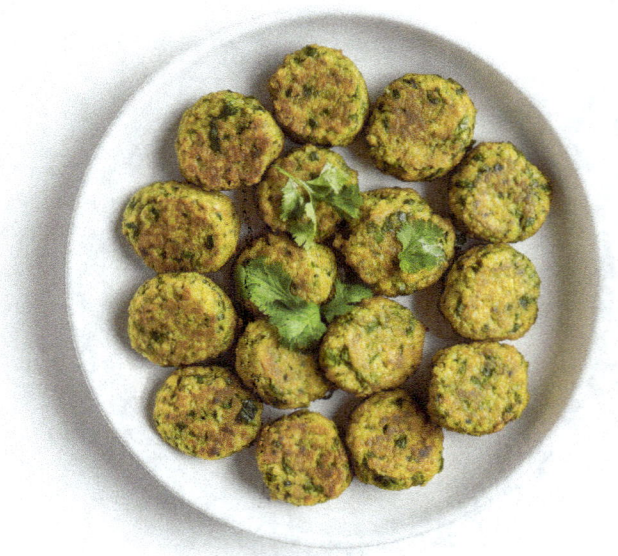

CHICKEN RAMEN BOWL

SERVES 2

PREP 15 min

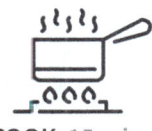

COOK 15 min

READY IN 30 min

INGREDIENTS

1 boneless, skinless chicken breast

6 ounces rice noodles

1 large egg

3 cups chicken broth

1 teaspoon coconut aminos

½ cup cabbage, sliced

½ cup carrots, shredded

¼ leek (white part only), chopped

½ teaspoon ginger powder

¼ teaspoon asafoetida (optional)

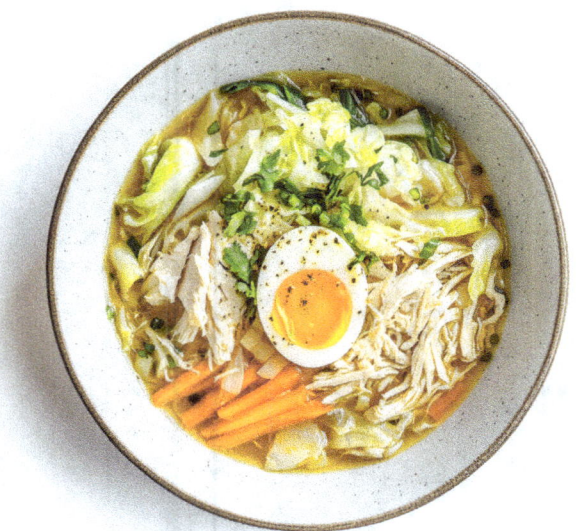

DIRECTIONS

1. Cover the egg in a medium saucepan with enough water to submerge it by 1 inch. Bring to a boil, then remove from heat. Cover and let sit for 7 minutes for a soft-set egg, or longer for a hard-boiled egg. Remove the egg with tongs or a slotted spoon and submerge in a bowl of ice water to stop the cooking process. Once cooled, peel and halve the egg. Set aside.

2. Bring chicken broth and coconut aminos to a boil in a separate pot. Add the chicken breast and cook until thoroughly done, about 8-10 minutes. Remove the chicken, allow it to cool slightly, then shred with two forks. Return the shredded chicken to the broth.

3. Add the sliced cabbage, chopped leek, and shredded carrots to the pot with the chicken broth and shredded chicken. Simmer for about 3-5 minutes until the vegetables are tender.

4. Add rice noodles to the pot. Cook according to the package instructions, usually about 3-5 minutes. Adjust the broth quantity as necessary, adding more chicken broth or water to ensure the noodles are submerged. Season with ginger powder, asafoetida, and salt to taste.

5. Remove the soup from heat. Serve the ramen warm, garnishing each bowl with a half of the cooked egg.

PER SERVING (about 2 cups) Calories: 272: Total fat: 5g; Protein: 24g; Carbohydrates: 27g; Fiber: 2g

THAI CHICKEN WRAPS

SERVES 4

PREP 20 min

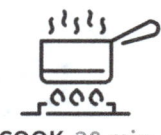
COOK 20 min

READY IN 40 min

INGREDIENTS

1 skinless chicken breast, cut into strips or cubed

1 ½ tablespoons olive oil, divided

1 cup cabbage, finely shredded

1 medium carrot, shredded

¼ teaspoon asafoetida

4 gluten-free tortillas (or see recipe on p. 164)

Salt to taste

Peanut Sauce:

2 tablespoons creamy peanut butter (no added sugar or oils)

¼ cup coconut aminos

1 tablespoon maple syrup

1 teaspoon sesame oil (optional)

¼ teaspoon ground ginger

3 tablespoons fresh cilantro, chopped

DIRECTIONS

1. In a skillet over medium heat, add 1 tablespoon olive oil. Once hot, add the chicken and sprinkle the asafoetida on top. Stir to coat and cook until the chicken reaches an internal temperature of 165°F. Season with salt to taste.

2. While the chicken is cooking, whisk together all the peanut sauce ingredients (peanut butter, coconut aminos, maple syrup, sesame oil, ginger, and cilantro) in a small bowl until smooth and well-blended. Set aside.

3. In the same pan, add the remaining ½ tablespoon of olive oil over medium-high heat. Add the shredded cabbage and carrot, stir-frying for 2-3 minutes until the vegetables are crisp-tender.

4. Place a gluten-free tortilla on a plate. Add the cooked chicken and stir-fried cabbage-carrot mixture. Drizzle with the prepared peanut sauce. Optionally, garnish with fresh basil or chopped peanuts for added crunch and flavor.

5. Wrap the tortilla around the fillings and serve the wraps cold or at room temperature. Enjoy!

PER SERVING (1 wrap) Calories: 220; Total fat: 9g; Protein: 12g; Carbohydrates: 20g; Fiber: 3g

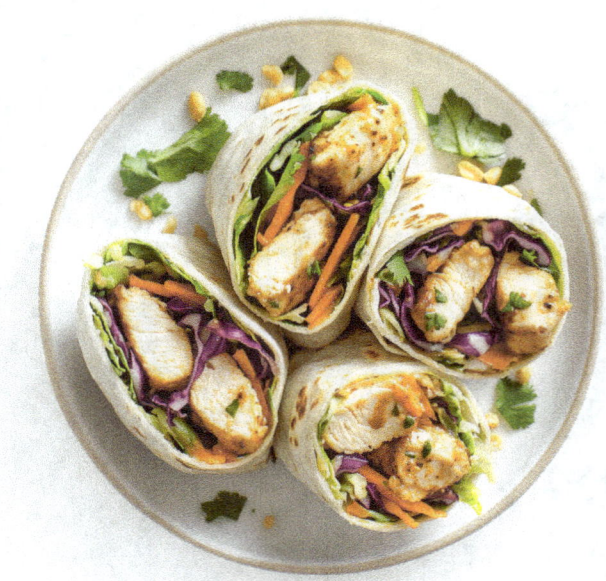

FISH TACOS

 **SERVES** 4

 **PREP** 15 min

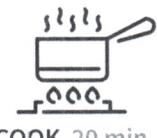 **COOK** 20 min

 **READY IN** 35 min

INGREDIENTS

1 pound (16 oz.) white fish fillets (such as cod or tilapia)

1 tablespoon olive oil, divided

½ teaspoon ground cumin

½ teaspoon dried oregano

½ teaspoon sweet paprika (optional, if tolerated)

¼ teaspoon salt (or to taste)

1 tablespoon fresh lime zest (optional)

1 cup purple and green cabbage, shredded

4 gluten-free tortillas (or see recipe on p. 165)

2 tablespoons fresh cilantro, chopped

Avocado sauce for dressing (optional, see recipe on p. 170)

DIRECTIONS

1. Pat the fish fillets dry and season both sides with cumin, oregano, paprika (if using), and salt. Sprinkle lime zest over the fillets for a burst of citrus flavor.

2. Heat ½ tablespoon of olive oil in a non-stick skillet over medium heat. Once the oil is hot, add the fish fillets and cook for 3-4 minutes per side, or until the fish is cooked through and flakes easily with a fork. Remove from the pan and set aside.

3. In the same skillet, add the remaining ½ tablespoon of olive oil. Add the shredded cabbage and sauté over medium heat for 5-7 minutes, stirring occasionally until the cabbage is softened but still has a bit of texture. Season with a pinch of salt if needed.

4. Warm the tortillas in a dry skillet over medium heat for about 30 seconds on each side, or until they are soft and pliable.

5. Break the cooked fish into smaller pieces and divide it among the tortillas. Top each taco with a generous portion of the sautéed cabbage and drizzle with the avocado sauce.

6. Sprinkle fresh cilantro on top of the tacos and serve immediately.

PER SERVING (1 taco) Calories: 210; Total fat: 5g; Protein: 26g
Carbohydrates: 10g; Fiber: 2g

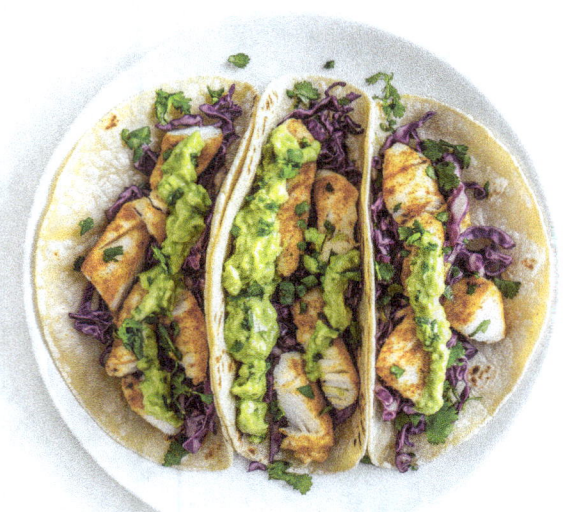

KOREAN RICE BOWL

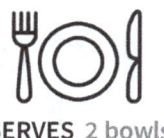
SERVES 2 bowls

PREP 20 min

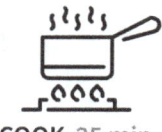
COOK 25 min

READY IN 45 min

INGREDIENTS

⅓ pound lean ground turkey (about ⅔ cup)

1 egg, beaten

1 medium carrot, cut into matchsticks

1 small beet, peeled and shredded (squeeze out excess moisture for crunch)

1 cup spinach, rinsed

Pinch of asafoetida (optional)

1 teaspoon salt, more to taste

1 cup cooked white rice

1 teaspoon sesame oil, plus more for cooking

3 teaspoons coconut aminos

½ teaspoon fresh ginger, grated

2 teaspoons maple syrup

Sesame seeds (optional, for maintenance phase)

PER SERVING (1 medium bowl)
Calories: 335; Total fat: 7g; Protein: 30g; Carbohydrates: 35g; Fiber: 2g

DIRECTIONS

1. In a small bowl, mix coconut aminos, ginger, maple syrup, and sesame oil. Set aside.

2. Heat a drizzle of oil in a medium skillet over medium heat. Cook the ground turkey until no pink remains. Add the prepared sauce and simmer for about 5 minutes until thickened.

3. In the same skillet, add a bit more sesame oil. Add carrots with a pinch of salt. Sauté for 3-5 minutes until tender but still crunchy. Remove and set aside.

4. Add more sesame oil to the skillet. Add shredded beet with a pinch of salt. Sauté for about 5 minutes until slightly soft. Remove and set aside with carrots.

5. Add spinach to the skillet with a bit of sesame oil and asafoetida. Cook until wilted, about 5 minutes. Season with salt and set aside.

6. Clean the skillet, add a drizzle of oil, and pour in the beaten egg. Cook until set, about 4-5 minutes. Flip and cook the other side for another 2-3 minutes. Season with salt and cut into strips.

7. Divide cooked rice between two bowls. Top with cooked turkey, sautéed carrots, beets, spinach, and egg strips. Garnish with sesame seeds if desired.

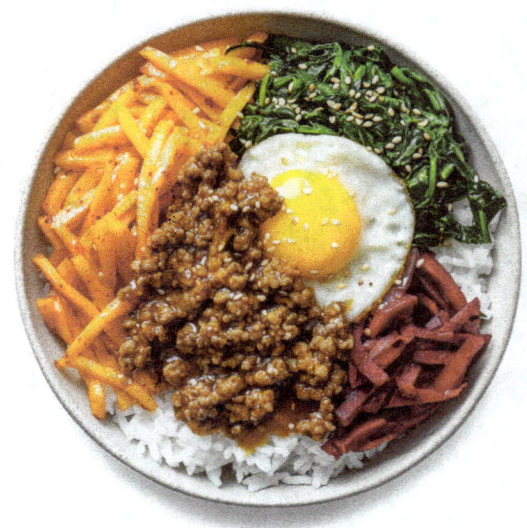

CREAMY CHICKEN KALE SOUP

SERVES 4

PREP 20 min

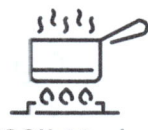
COOK 30 min

READY IN 50 min

INGREDIENTS

1 boneless, skinless chicken breast

1-2 cups kale, roughly chopped

1 ½ cups carrots, peeled and diced

1 ½ cups celery, diced

8 ounces baby bella mushrooms, sliced (about 3 cups)

5 cups chicken or vegetable broth

1 tablespoon fresh thyme

2-3 tablespoons arrowroot flour or potato starch

⅓ cup lite coconut milk

1 teaspoon olive oil

Salt to taste

DIRECTIONS

1. Heat the olive oil in a large Dutch oven or stockpot over medium-high heat. Add the diced carrots and celery, season with a pinch of salt, and sauté for about 3 minutes until they begin to soften. Add the fresh thyme and sliced mushrooms, giving everything a quick toss.

2. Pour in the chicken or vegetable broth, then add the chicken breast to the pot. Bring the soup to a boil, then reduce the heat to a simmer. Cover the pot with a lid and cook for about 15-20 minutes, or until the vegetables are tender and the chicken is fully cooked through.

3. While the soup is simmering, in a medium bowl, mix together the potato starch or arrowroot flour, coconut milk, and ¼ cup of water until smooth. Use a whisk or blender to remove any lumps. Set aside.

4. Once the chicken is cooked through, remove it from the pot and shred it using two forks. Return the shredded chicken to the pot.

5. Slowly pour the arrowroot/coconut milk mixture into the soup, stirring constantly. Let it simmer for a few minutes until the soup thickens slightly.

6. Stir in the chopped kale and allow the soup to simmer for another 3-5 minutes until the kale wilts and the soup is heated through.

7. Taste the soup and add more salt if needed. Serve warm and enjoy!

PER SERVING (about 1 ½ cups) Calories: 117; Total fat: 3g; Protein: 11g; Carbohydrates: 8g; Fiber: 3g

TURKEY QUINOA MEATLOAF

SERVES 4

PREP 30 min

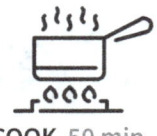
COOK 50 min

READY IN 1 h 20 min

INGREDIENTS

1 pound lean ground turkey (about 2 cups)

¼ cup uncooked quinoa, rinsed

½ cup chicken broth or water

2 eggs, beaten

1 tablespoon olive oil

1 small carrot, grated

¼ cup leek (white part only), finely chopped

1 teaspoon fresh thyme, minced

1 teaspoon fresh rosemary, minced

½ teaspoon ground cumin

¼ teaspoon ground oregano

1 teaspoon salt

PER SERVING (¼ of the meatloaf)
Calories: 286; Total fat: 9g; Protein: 40g; Carbohydrates: 8g; Fiber: 1g

DIRECTIONS

1. In a small saucepan over medium-high heat, combine the quinoa and chicken broth. Bring to a simmer, then reduce heat to medium-low, cover, and cook until the quinoa is tender and the broth has been absorbed, about 15 to 20 minutes. Remove from heat and let cool slightly.

2. Preheat the oven to 350°F with a rack in the center position. Line a large rimmed baking sheet with parchment paper.

3. Heat the olive oil in a large skillet over medium heat. Add the leek and carrot, and sauté until the leek is softened and translucent, about 5 minutes. Remove from heat.

4. In a large bowl, combine the ground turkey, cooked quinoa, sautéed vegetables, eggs, cumin, thyme, rosemary, oregano, and salt. Mix well until thoroughly combined.

5. With wet hands, form the mixture into a loaf shape on the prepared baking sheet. Bake for about 50 minutes, or until the internal temperature reaches 165°F on a meat thermometer.

6. Let the meatloaf rest for 10 minutes after baking. Slice and serve warm.

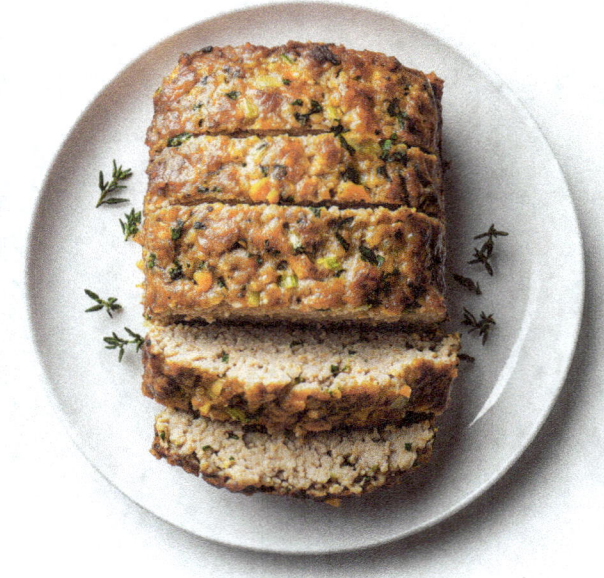

GRILLED SHRIMP SKEWERS

SERVES 4

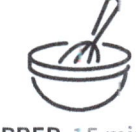
PREP 15 min

COOK 8 min

READY IN 50 min

INGREDIENTS

1 pound large shrimp, peeled and deveined (about 1 ¾ cups)

2 zucchinis, cut into chunks

2 tablespoons olive oil

6-8 button mushrooms, halved

½ teaspoon ground cumin

1 teaspoon dried oregano

1 tablespoon fresh basil, minced

Zest of 1 lemon

½ teaspoon salt

DIRECTIONS

1. In a large shallow dish, combine the olive oil, cumin, oregano, fresh basil, lemon zest, and salt. Stir to mix well.

2. Thread the shrimp, zucchini chunks, and halved mushrooms onto wooden skewers, alternating ingredients for variety.

3. Place the assembled skewers into the dish with the marinade, making sure they are well-coated. Cover and refrigerate for at least 30 minutes to allow the flavors to meld.

4. Preheat your grill to medium-high heat. Lightly grease the grill grates to prevent sticking.

5. Remove the shrimp skewers from the marinade, discarding any excess marinade. Place the skewers on the hot grill and cook for about 3 minutes on each side, or until the shrimp are pink and fully cooked.

6. Serve the grilled shrimp skewers immediately and enjoy with your favorite side dish!

NOTE

- Soak wooden skewers in water for 20-30 minutes prior to grilling to prevent burning.

PER SERVING (2 skewers) Calories: 216; Total fat: 9g; Protein: 27g; Carbohydrates: 4g; Fiber: 1g

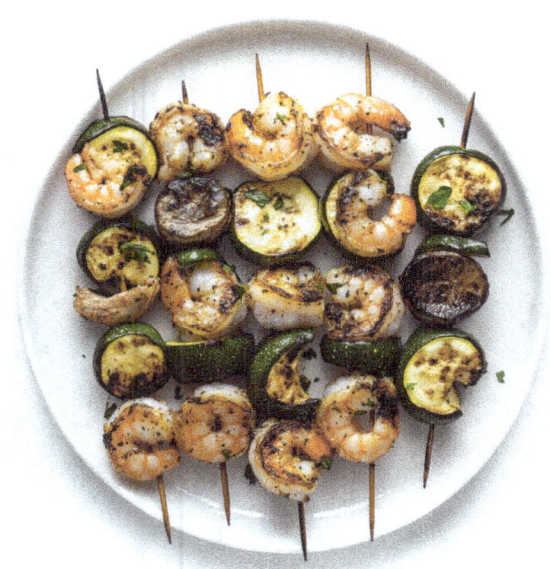

BUTTERNUT SQUASH PASTA

SERVES 2   **PREP** 10 min   **COOK** 15 min   **READY IN** 25 min

INGREDIENTS

½ cup butternut squash, peeled and diced

1 medium carrot, peeled and chopped

2 tablespoons canned coconut milk

1 tablespoon nutritional yeast

½ teaspoon dried or fresh dill

A pinch of asafoetida (optional)

A small dash of liquid aminos or coconut aminos (optional, adjust to taste)

6 ounces gluten-free pasta of your choice

Salt to taste

DIRECTIONS

1. Bring a large pot of water to a boil. Add your pasta and cook according to the package directions until al dente. Reserve ¼ cup of the pasta water, then drain the pasta and set it aside.

2. While the pasta is cooking, bring another small pot of water to a boil. Add the chopped carrot and butternut squash. Boil until they are soft and tender, about 10-12 minutes.

3. Once the vegetables are cooked, transfer them to a blender or food processor. Add the coconut milk, reserved pasta water, nutritional yeast, dried dill, asafoetida, and liquid aminos. Blend until smooth and creamy. Adjust the consistency with more pasta water if needed.

4. Pour the sauce into a pan and simmer for 2-3 minutes over low heat. Taste and adjust seasoning with salt or more liquid aminos if necessary.

5. Add the cooked pasta to the sauce and toss to combine. Serve warm and enjoy!

PER SERVING (about 1 ½ cups)
Calories: 181; Total fat: 4g; Protein: 9g;
Carbohydrates: 20g; Fiber: 5g

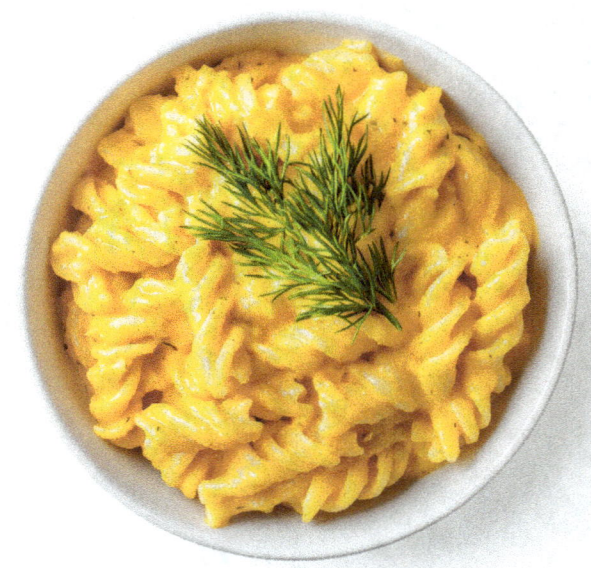

CHICKEN LENTIL STEW

 **SERVES** 3

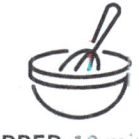 **PREP** 10 min

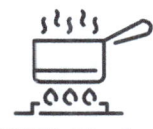 **COOK** 35 min

 **READY IN** 45 min

INGREDIENTS

½ cup dry red lentils, rinsed

½ pound lean ground chicken (about 1 cup)

2 cups chicken broth or water

½ leek (white part only), chopped

1 medium carrot, peeled and diced

1 ½ tablespoons olive oil

¼ teaspoon asafoetida (optional)

½ tablespoon dried thyme

½ teaspoon ground cumin

¼ teaspoon ground coriander

Salt to taste

DIRECTIONS

1. Heat olive oil in a large pot over medium heat. Add the ground chicken and cook, breaking it apart until browned and cooked through.

2. Add the chopped leek and diced carrot to the pot. Sauté for 3-4 minutes until the vegetables soften slightly.

3. Stir in the thyme, cumin, coriander, and asafoetida (if using). Cook for 1 minute until fragrant.

4. Add the red lentils and pour in the chicken broth or water. Bring to a boil, then reduce to a simmer. Cover and cook for 20-25 minutes, until the lentils are tender and the stew has thickened. Stir occasionally.

5. Taste and adjust seasoning with salt if needed. Serve warm and enjoy!

PER SERVING (about 1 cup) Calories: 207; Total fat: 10g; Protein: 18g; Carbohydrates: 8g; Fiber: 2g

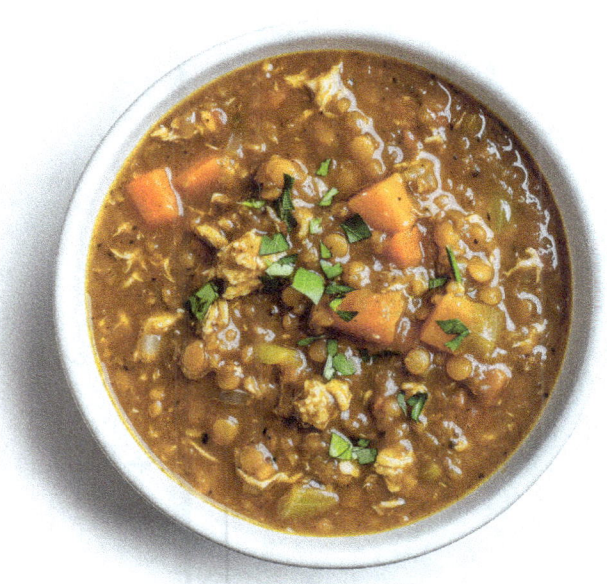

PAN-SEARED SEA BASS

 **SERVES** 2

 **PREP** 5 min

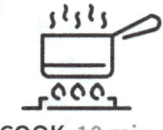 **COOK** 10 min

 **READY IN** 15 min

INGREDIENTS

2 sea bass fillets, with or without skin

1 tablespoon olive oil

¼ teaspoon salt

¼ teaspoon asafoetida (optional)

½ tablespoon ghee (optional, for maintenance phase)

Zest of 1 lemon

Fresh cilantro for garnish (optional)

DIRECTIONS

1. Pat dry the sea bass fillets with paper towels. Season both sides of the fish with asafoetida, salt, and lemon zest.

2. Heat a cast iron skillet over medium-high heat. Add the olive oil and ghee (if using), and heat until melted and hot.

3. Place the sea bass fillets in the hot skillet. Cook for about 4 minutes, until the edges are golden and crispy. Flip the fillets carefully and cook for another 4-5 minutes, or until the fish is flaky and cooked through.

4. Garnish with a sprig of cilantro and sprinkle additional lemon zest for brightness.

PER SERVING (1 sea bass fillet)
Calories: 185; Total fat: 9g; Protein: 23g;
Carbohydrates: 0g; Fiber: 0g

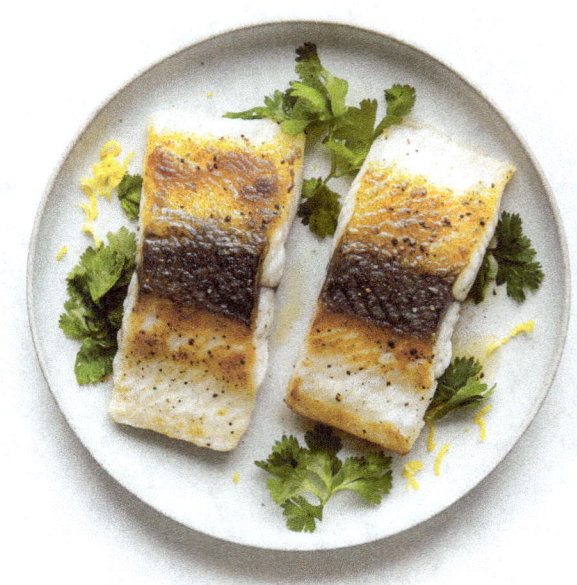

VEGETABLES PATTIES

SERVES 4

PREP 15 min

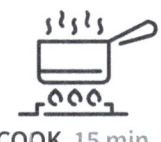
COOK 15 min

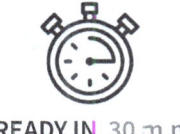
READY IN 30 min

INGREDIENTS

3 cups fresh baby spinach, finely chopped

2 tablespoons olive oil, divided

1 medium parsnip, peeled and grated

½ cup carrot, peeled and grated

¼ leek (white part only), thinly sliced and rinsed

¼ cup Kalamata or black olives, finely diced (optional)

2 eggs, beaten

¼ cup coconut or almond flour

½ teaspoon ground cumin

1 teaspoon dried oregano

½ teaspoon salt

DIRECTIONS

1. In a medium skillet, heat 1 tablespoon of olive oil over medium heat. Add the leek and cook until soft, about 3-4 minutes. Stir in the spinach and cook until wilted. Remove from heat and transfer to a large mixing bowl.

2. To the same bowl, add the grated parsnip, grated carrot, diced olives (if using), cumin, oregano, and salt. Stir to combine well.

3. Pour the beaten eggs into the vegetable mixture, followed by the coconut or almond flour. Mix until the ingredients are well incorporated and can hold together.

4. Shape the mixture into patties, about ½ inch thick and 2-3 inches wide.

5. Heat the remaining tablespoon of olive oil in the same skillet over medium heat. When the oil is hot, add the patties and cook for 5-7 minutes on each side, or until golden brown and crispy.

6. Serve the patties warm and enjoy as a light meal or side dish.

PER SERVING (2 patties) Calories: 133; Total fat: 7g; Protein: 5g; Carbohydrates: 7g; Fiber: 5g

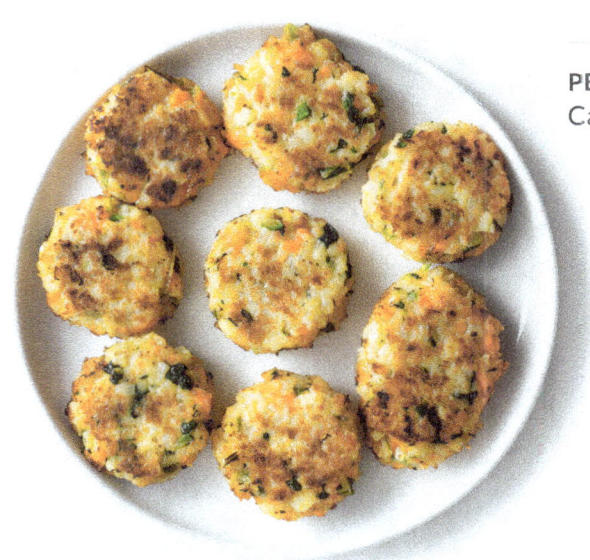

GRILLED ZA'ATAR CHICKEN TENDERS

SERVES 4

PREP 10 min

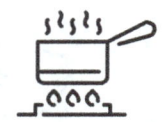

COOK 20-30 min

READY IN 2 h 40 min

INGREDIENTS

1 pound chicken tenderloins (about 2 cups)

1 tablespoon olive oil

1 teaspoon water

¼ teaspoon dried thyme (or substitute oregano)

½ teaspoon ground turmeric

½ teaspoon cumin

¼ teaspoon ground coriander

¼ teaspoon toasted sesame seeds

¼ teaspoon sumac

½ teaspoon salt

Fresh cilantro, for garnish (optional)

DIRECTIONS

1. In a small bowl, mix the olive oil, water, thyme (or oregano), turmeric, cumin, coriander, sesame seeds, sumac, and salt to form a paste.

2. Place the chicken tenderloins in a resealable quart-sized bag. Add the spice paste, seal the bag, and shake it to coat the chicken evenly. Refrigerate for 2-3 hours to allow the flavors to infuse.

3. Preheat your grill or grill skillet to medium-high heat. Clean and oil the grill grates to prevent sticking.

4. Once the grill is hot, add the chicken tenderloins in batches. Cook for 7-10 minutes per batch, or until the internal temperature reaches 165°F, ensuring the chicken is cooked through. Depending on your grill size, you may need to do this in two or three batches.

5. Serve the grilled chicken with your desired side dish. Garnish with fresh cilantro for a burst of flavor.

PER SERVING (3 chicken tenders)
Calories: 140; Total fat: 4g; Protein: 26g;
Carbohydrates: 0g; Fiber: 0g

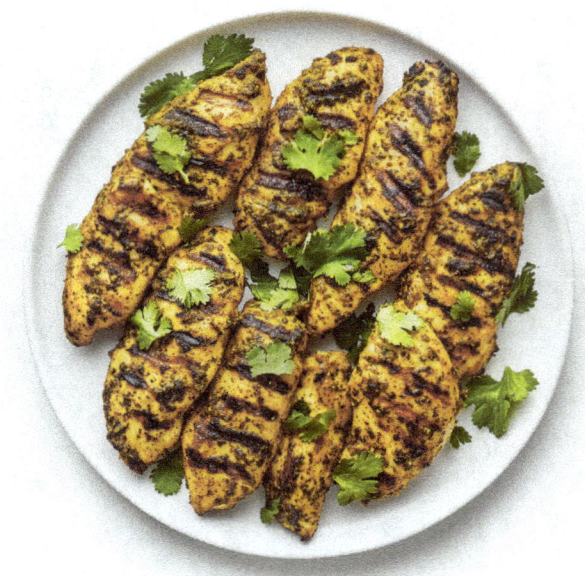

SWEDISH MEATBALLS

SERVES 4

PREP 20 min

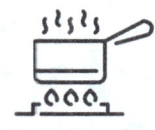
COOK 50 min

READY IN 1 h 10 min

INGREDIENTS

1 pound lean ground turkey (about 2 cups)

1 large egg

½ cup gluten-free breadcrumbs

1 tablespoon parsley, minced

½ teaspoon asafoetida (optional)

1 teaspoon coconut aminos

½ teaspoon dried oregano

Mushroom Sauce:

1 cup mushrooms, sliced

½ leek (white part only), diced

2 cups chicken broth

¼ cup canned coconut milk

1 tablespoon olive oil

½ tablespoon liquid aminos or coconut aminos

2 tablespoons potato starch or arrowroot flour

¼ teaspoon salt

DIRECTIONS

1. Preheat your oven to 400°F.

2. In a large bowl, mix together the ground turkey, egg, gluten-free breadcrumbs, minced parsley, asafoetida, 1 teaspoon liquid aminos, and dried oregano.

3. Form the mixture into 12-15 meatballs and place them on a parchment-lined baking sheet.

4. Bake for 17-20 minutes, or until the internal temperature reaches 155°F and the meatballs are browned on top.

5. In a small bowl, whisk together 1/2 cup of the chicken broth with the potato starch (or arrowroot flour) until smooth. Set aside.

6. In a large skillet over medium heat, heat the olive oil. Add the mushrooms and diced leek, and cook until the mushrooms are tender and the leek is translucent, about 4-5 minutes.

7. Pour the remaining chicken broth into the skillet, along with the broth and starch mixture, the coconut milk, and 1/2 tablespoon of liquid aminos. Bring the sauce to a simmer, stirring frequently until it thickens slightly.

8. Add the baked meatballs to the simmering sauce. Let them cook in the sauce for another 10 minutes, until the meatballs reach an internal temperature of 165°F and are fully cooked through.

9. Serve the meatballs with the sauce over a side of your choice, and enjoy!

PER SERVING (4 meatballs) Calories: 245; Total fat: 4g; Protein: 38g; Carbohydrates: 12g; Fiber: 0g

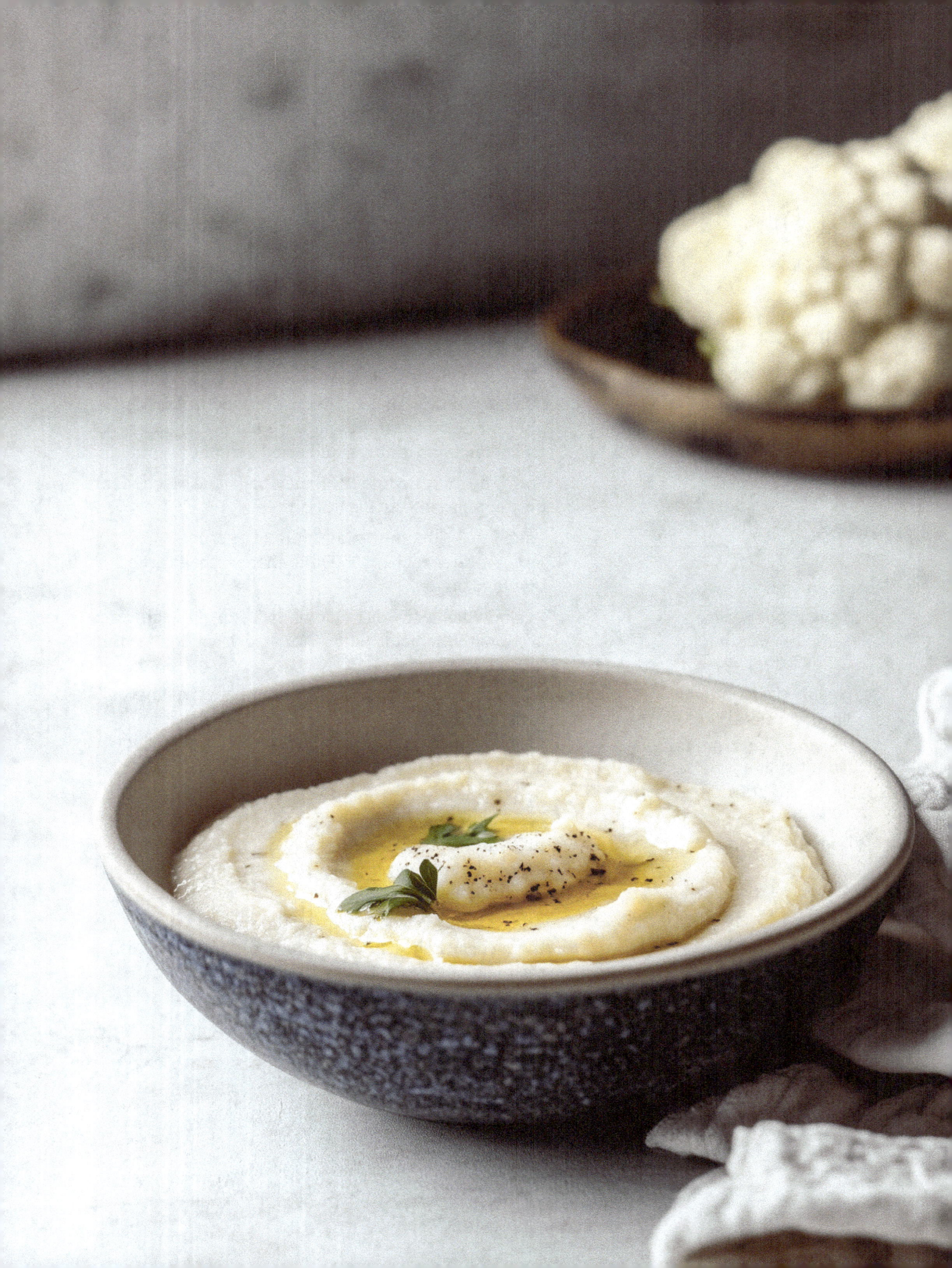

CHAPTER SIX

SIDE DISHES

MASHED RUTABAGA

  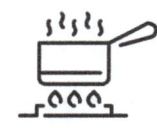 

SERVES 2   **PREP** 10 min   **COOK** 30 min   **READY IN** 40 min

INGREDIENTS

2 medium rutabagas, peeled and chopped into 1-inch chunks

1 tablespoon olive oil

½ teaspoon salt, plus more to taste

1 tablespoon chopped parsley for garnish (optional)

DIRECTIONS

1. In a large saucepan, add the rutabaga chunks and enough water to cover them by about 1 inch. Stir in ½ teaspoon of salt.

2. Bring the water to a boil over high heat, then reduce the heat to medium and simmer the rutabaga until it is tender, which typically takes about 25 to 35 minutes.

3. Once the rutabaga is tender, drain the water and return the rutabaga to the saucepan.

4. Add the olive oil to the cooked rutabaga. Use a fork or potato masher to mash the rutabaga to your desired consistency.

5. Taste the mashed rutabaga and add additional salt if needed.

6. Serve the mashed rutabaga warm, garnished with chopped parsley.

PER SERVING (about 1 cup)
Calories: 202; Total fat: 7g; Protein: 4g;
Carbohydrates: 24g; Fiber: 9g

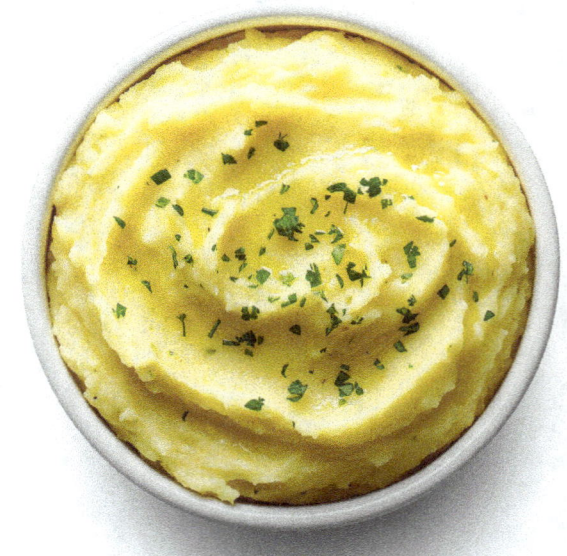

MUSHROOM RICE

SERVES 2

PREP 5 min

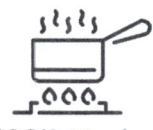
COOK 20 min

READY IN 30 min

INGREDIENTS

6 ounces mushrooms, sliced (about 2 ⅓ cups)

1 cup uncooked white rice

2 cups vegetable or chicken broth (or water)

1 teaspoon olive oil

6-8 sprigs thyme, leaves stripped

Salt to taste

DIRECTIONS

1. In a saucepan, heat the olive oil over medium-high heat. Add the sliced mushrooms and sauté for about 4 to 5 minutes until they begin to brown. Season with salt and thyme leaves during the last minute of cooking.

2. Remove half of the sautéed mushrooms from the saucepan and set them aside for later use.

3. In the same saucepan, add the rice and broth. Bring the mixture to a boil, then reduce the heat to low. Cover and simmer for 10-15 minutes, or until the rice is cooked and all the broth has been absorbed.

4. Stir the reserved mushrooms back into the cooked rice. Adjust the seasoning with additional salt and thyme if needed.

5. Fluff the rice with a fork before serving to separate the grains and integrate the mushrooms evenly. Serve warm as a side dish or a light main course.

PER SERVING (about 1 cup) Calories: 376; Total fat: 3g; Protein: 9g; Carbohydrates: 73g; Fiber: 2g

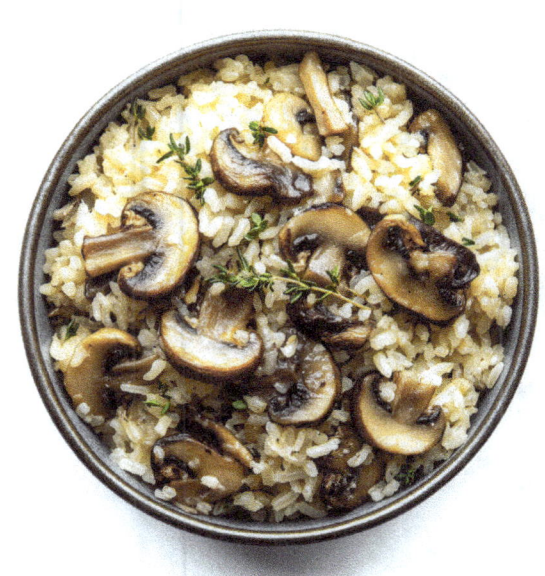

ROASTED BROCCOLI

SERVES 2

PREP 10 min

COOK 20 min

READY IN 30 min

INGREDIENTS

8 ounces broccoli, cut into florets (about 2 ½ cups)

2 teaspoons olive oil

Salt to taste

¼ cup dairy-free parmesan cheese (optional, for maintenance phase; see p. 175)

DIRECTIONS

1. Set your oven to 400 degrees F. Line a baking sheet with parchment paper or lightly grease it with oil.

2. In a bowl, toss the broccoli florets with olive oil and a pinch of salt until evenly coated.

3. Spread the broccoli florets in a single layer on the prepared baking sheet. Roast in the oven for 15 to 22 minutes, or until the edges are nicely browned.

4. Remove the broccoli from the oven and immediately sprinkle with dairy-free parmesan cheese, if using.

PER SERVING (about 1 cup)
Calories: 78; Total fat: 5g; Protein: 3g;
Carbohydrates: 4g; Fiber: 3g

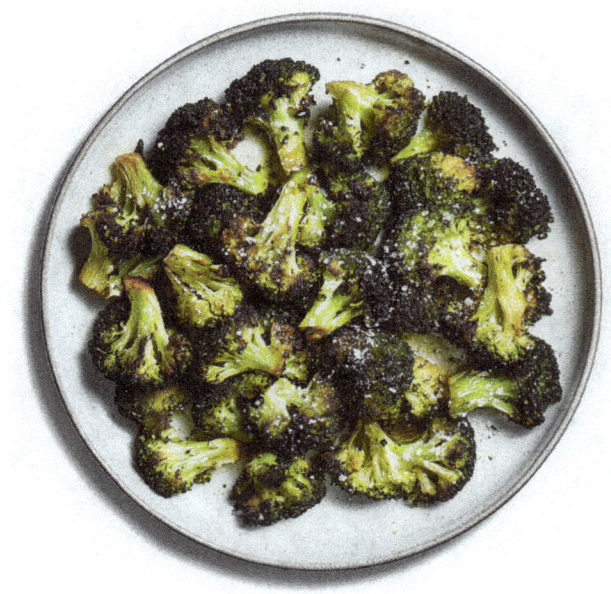

SAUTÉED BRUSSELS SPROUTS

SERVES 2

PREP 10 min

COOK 10 min

READY IN 20 min

INGREDIENTS

6 ounces Brussels sprouts, shredded or julienned (about 2 cups)

1 tablespoon olive oil

½ teaspoon asafoetida (optional)

½ teaspoon salt

¼ cup dairy-free Parmesan cheese (optional, for maintenance phase; see p. 175)

DIRECTIONS

1. In a non-stick skillet over medium-high heat, add the olive oil. Swirl the skillet to coat the bottom with oil once it's hot and shining.

2. Add the shredded Brussels sprouts, asafoetida, and salt to the skillet. Cook for 6 to 8 minutes, stirring occasionally, until the sprouts are evenly browned and just tender inside.

3. Remove the skillet from the heat. If using, toss the cooked Brussels sprouts with the dairy-free Parmesan cheese.

4. Enjoy the Brussels sprouts warm as a side dish, offering a tasty blend of nutty and slightly sweet flavors enhanced by the optional cheese.

PER SERVING (1 cup approx.) Calories: 96; Total fat: 7g; Protein: 3g; Carbohydrates: 4g; Fiber: 3g

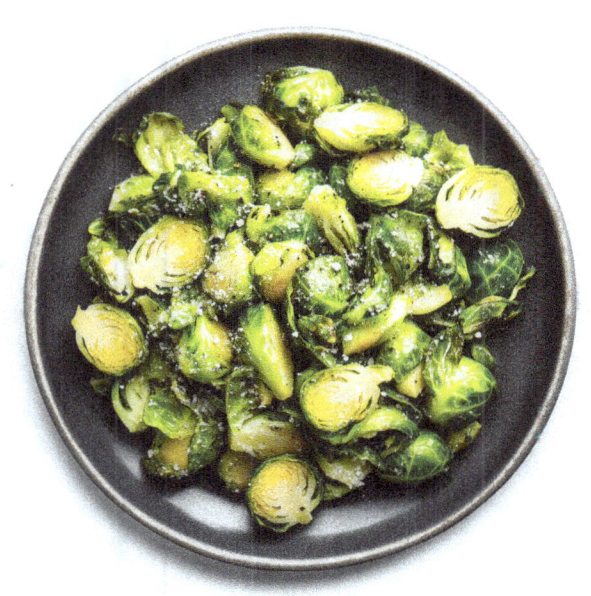

MUSHROOM QUINOA PILAF

SERVES 2

PREP 15 min

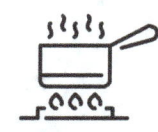

COOK 20 min

READY IN 35 min

INGREDIENTS

1 small carrot, peeled and shredded

½ cup quinoa, rinsed

1 cup vegetable broth

2 ounces mushrooms, stemmed and thinly sliced (about ¾ cup)

1 ½ tablespoons olive oil, divided

½ leek (white part only), thinly sliced and rinsed

¼ teaspoon asafoetida

2 tablespoons fresh parsley, chopped

½ teaspoon dried thyme

¼ cup pine nuts or pecans, chopped (optional)

Salt to taste

DIRECTIONS

1. In a medium saucepan, combine the quinoa and vegetable broth. Bring to a boil, then reduce heat to low, cover, and simmer until the quinoa is cooked and the liquid is absorbed, about 15 minutes.

2. While the quinoa cooks, heat 1 tablespoon of olive oil in a large skillet over medium heat. Add the shredded carrots, leeks, and thyme and cook for about 5 to 7 minutes until the carrots are tender.

3. Stir in the mushrooms and the remaining ½ tablespoon of olive oil to the skillet. Continue to cook, stirring frequently, until the mushrooms are tender and cooked through. Season with salt and asafoetida.

4. Add the cooked quinoa to the skillet with the vegetables. Stir in the chopped parsley and optional pine nuts or pecans. Taste and adjust seasoning if necessary. Serve warm.

PER SERVING (about 1 cup)
Calories: 275; Total fat: 12g; Protein: 7g; Carbohydrates: 29g; Fiber: 4g

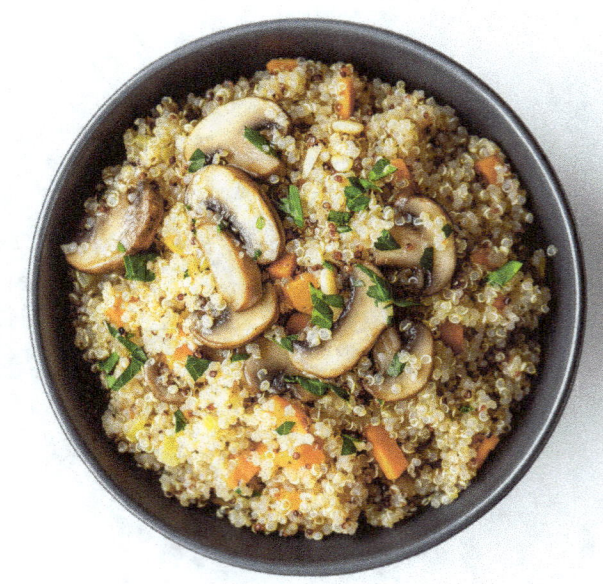

MASHED SWEET POTATOES

 **SERVES** 2

 **PREP** 10 min

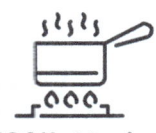 **COOK** 20 min

 **READY IN** 30 min

INGREDIENTS

2 medium sweet potatoes, peeled and cut into 1-inch pieces

½ cup unsweetened almond milk (or other plant-based milk)

1 teaspoon grated fresh ginger (optional)

½ teaspoon salt

DIRECTIONS

1. Place the sweet potatoes in a large saucepan and cover with at least 1-inch of water. Set over medium-high heat and bring to a boil.

2. Cover the saucepan with a lid and continue to boil until the sweet potatoes are tender, about 15-20 minutes.

3. Drain the water and return the sweet potatoes to the saucepan. Add the almond milk, grated ginger (if using), and salt. Use a potato masher to mash the mixture until smooth.

4. Stir the mashed sweet potatoes well to ensure all ingredients are evenly mixed.

5. Serve the mashed sweet potatoes immediately, perfect as a side dish for festive meals or everyday dinners.

PER SERVING (about 1 cup) Calories: 109; Total fat: 1g; Protein: 2g; Carbohydrates: 18g; Fiber: 4g

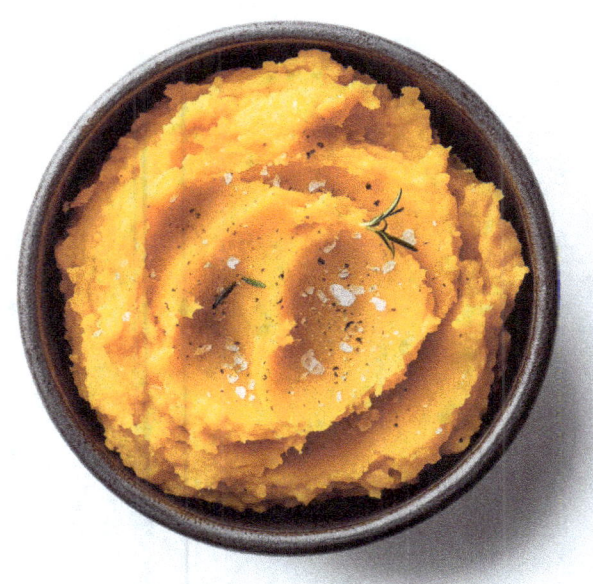

KALE COCONUT "FRIED" RICE

SERVES 4

PREP 15 min

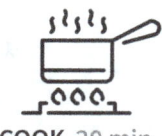
COOK 20 min

READY IN 35 min

INGREDIENTS

1 bunch kale, stems removed and leaves finely shredded

½ cup unsweetened coconut flakes

2 cups cooked white rice

1 cup carrots, thinly sliced

2 tablespoons fresh parsley, chopped

1 egg, beaten

1 egg white

½ teaspoon asafoetida (optional)

2 teaspoons coconut oil, divided

1 tablespoon coconut aminos

¼ teaspoon salt

Fresh cilantro (optional, for garnish)

PER SERVING (about 1 cup)
Calories: 231; Total fat: 10g; Protein: 5g; Carbohydrates: 26g; Fiber: 3g

DIRECTIONS

1. Heat 1 teaspoon of coconut oil in a wok or non-stick skillet over medium-high heat. Add the eggs and cook, stirring occasionally, until scrambled and lightly set. Transfer the eggs to a bowl and set aside. Wipe out the skillet with a paper towel if necessary.

2. Add the remaining teaspoon of coconut oil to the skillet. Stir in the parsley, kale, and carrots. Cook, stirring constantly, until the vegetables are tender and the kale is wilted, about 2-3 minutes. Season with salt and asafoetida during cooking. Transfer the cooked vegetables to the bowl with the scrambled eggs.

3. In the same skillet, add the coconut flakes and cook, stirring frequently, until lightly golden, about 1-2 minutes.

4. Add the cooked rice to the skillet with the toasted coconut flakes. Stir to combine and cook until the rice is thoroughly heated, about 3 minutes.

5. Return the eggs and vegetables to the skillet. Add the coconut aminos and stir everything together until well combined.

6. Divide the rice mixture among bowls. Garnish with fresh cilantro leaves if desired.

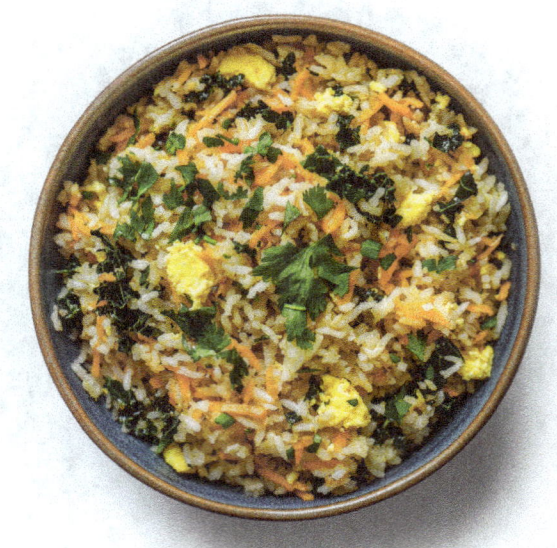

CREAMED SPINACH

SERVES 2

PREP 5 min

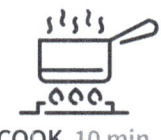
COOK 10 min

READY IN 15 min

INGREDIENTS

1 bunch spinach, stemmed and chopped

½ cup unsweetened almond milk

1 tablespoon olive oil

1 teaspoon potato starch or arrowroot flour

½ teaspoon salt

Pinch of ground nutmeg (optional, for maintenance phase)

DIRECTIONS

1. Heat the olive oil in a large pot over medium-high heat until shimmering. Add the chopped spinach, salt, and nutmeg (if using). Cook for about 3 minutes or until the spinach is wilted.

2. While the spinach cooks, whisk together the almond milk and potato starch or arrowroot flour in a small bowl. Pour this mixture over the wilted spinach.

3. Continue to cook, stirring constantly, until the sauce thickens, about 1 minute. Adjust the seasoning if necessary.

4. Serve the creamed spinach warm as a side dish to your favorite meals.

PER SERVING (about ½ cup) Calories: 112; Total fat: 8g; Protein: 5g; Carbohydrates: 3g; Fiber: 4g

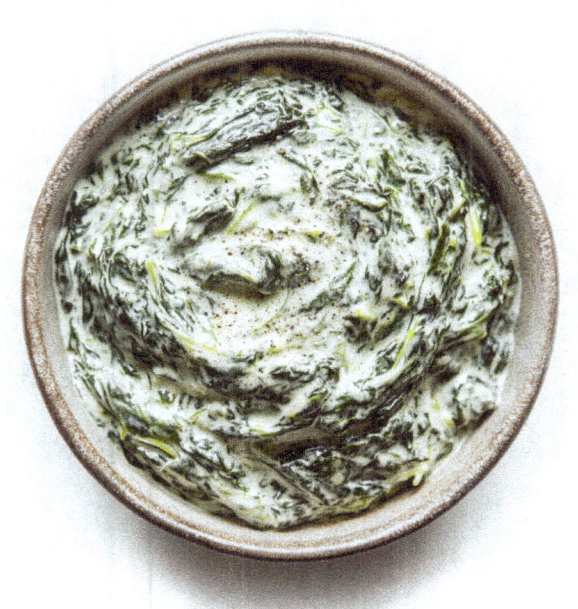

CAULIFLOWER PURÉE

SERVES 4

PREP 5 min

COOK 10-15 min

READY IN 15-20 min

INGREDIENTS

1 medium head cauliflower, cut into florets

2 tablespoons olive oil

1 teaspoon dried oregano

¼ teaspoon asafoetida (optional)

½ teaspoon salt, or to taste

DIRECTIONS

1. Add the cauliflower florets to a pot of boiling water and cook for 10-15 minutes, or until tender. Alternatively, steam the florets in a steamer basket over boiling water for the same time.

2. Drain the cauliflower thoroughly and let it sit for 2-3 minutes to allow excess moisture to evaporate. This step is key for a smooth, creamy purée rather than a watery one.

3. Transfer the cauliflower to a food processor or blender. Add the olive oil, herbs, asafoetida (if using), and salt. Blend until smooth and fluffy. Adjust the salt to taste.

4. Garnish with chopped fresh herbs and an additional drizzle of olive oil, if desired. Serve immediately and enjoy!

PER SERVING (about 1 cup)
Calories: 96; Total fat: 7g; Protein: 2g; Carbohydrates: 4g; Fiber: 3g

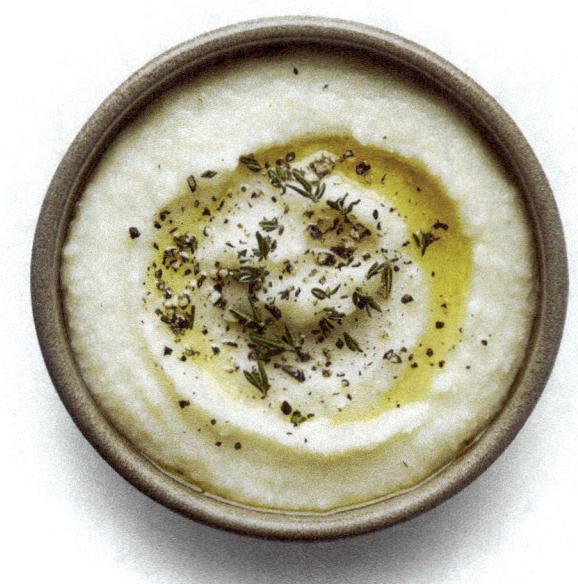

RICE LENTIL PILAF

 **SERVES** 4

 **PREP** 10 min

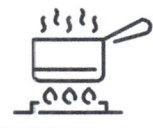 **COOK** 50 min

 **READY IN** 60 min

INGREDIENTS

½ cup brown lentils

½ cup uncooked basmati or long grain rice

1 tablespoon olive oil

¼ leek (white part only), chopped

1 cup vegetable broth (or water)

¼ teaspoon ground cumin

½ teaspoon ground coriander

¼ teaspoon ground turmeric (optional)

4 cups water

½ teaspoon salt

DIRECTIONS

1. In a large stock pot, bring 4 cups of water to a boil over high heat. Add the lentils and maintain a moderate boil for about 25 minutes, checking for doneness every few minutes after 20 minutes, until the lentils are just tender. Drain and set aside

2. Meanwhile, in a small saucepan, bring 1 cup of vegetable broth (or water) to a boil. Add the rice, cover, and reduce heat to a simmer. Cook for 20-25 minutes until the liquid has evaporated. Remove from heat and keep covered.

3. While the rice and lentils are cooking, heat the olive oil in a medium non-stick skillet over medium-high heat. Add the chopped leek, salt, cumin, coriander, and turmeric. Cook, stirring frequently, until the leek begins to soften and brown slightly.

4. Add the cooked lentils to the skillet with the leeks Then add the cooked rice and stir everything together until well blended.

5. Adjust seasoning if necessary and serve the pilaf warm.

PER SERVING (about ¾ cup) Calories: 202; Total fat: 4g; Protein: 7g; Carbohydrates: 31g; Fiber: 3g

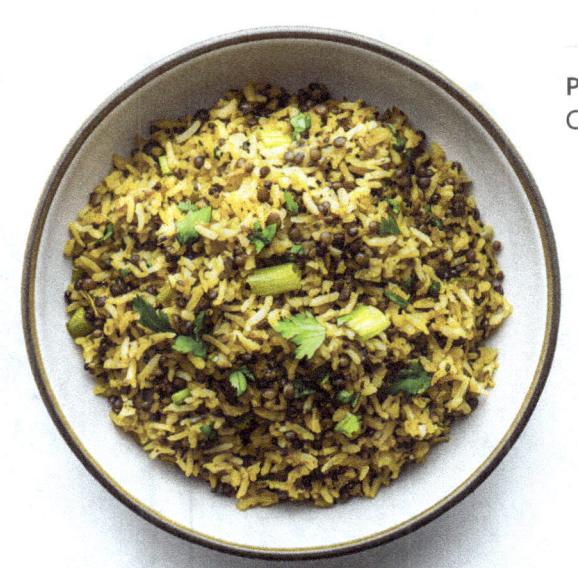

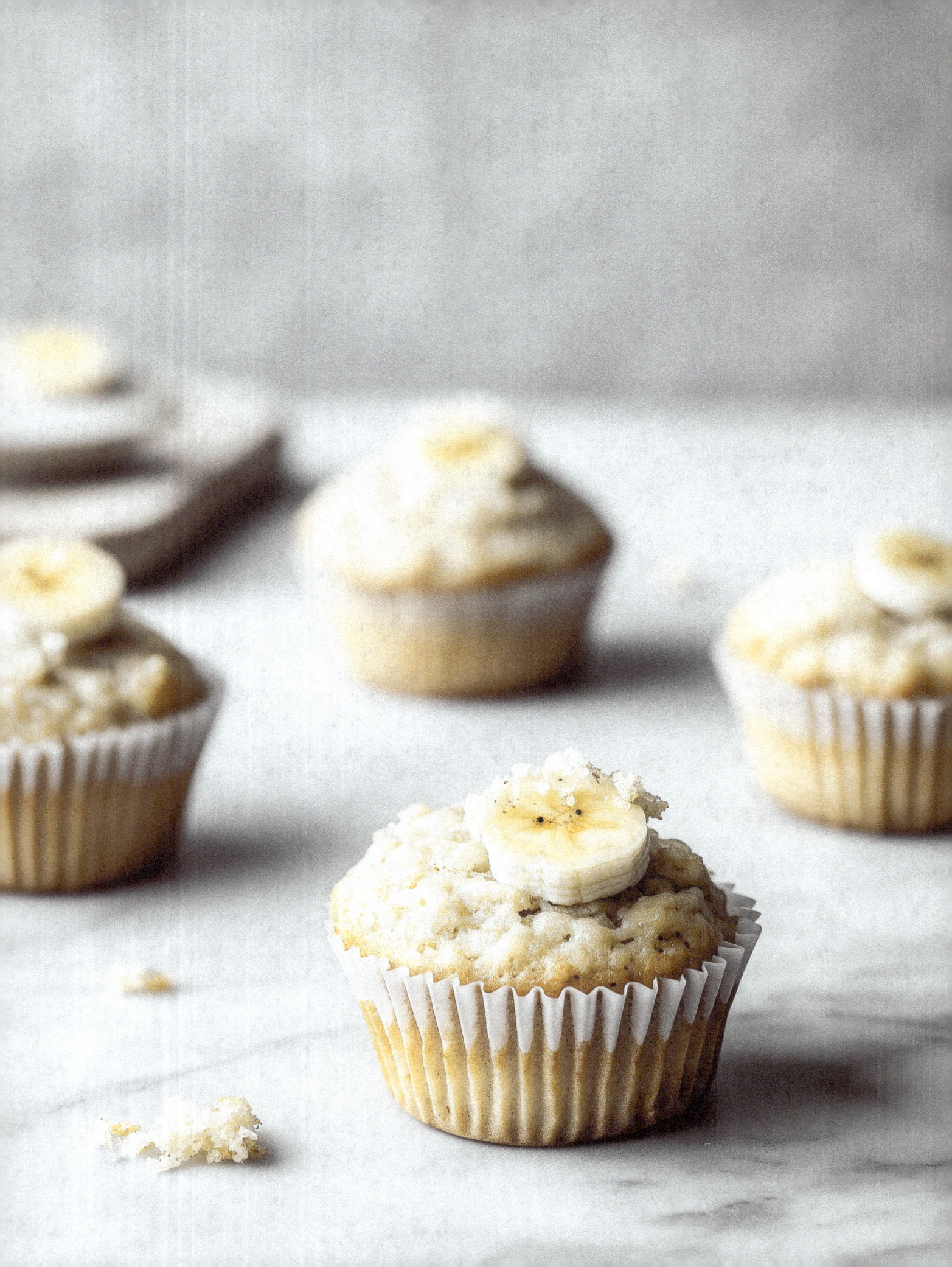

CHAPTER SEVEN

SNACKS & SWEETS

BAKED ZUCCHINI FRIES

SERVES 2

PREP 10 min

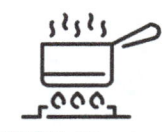
COOK 20 min

READY IN 30 min

INGREDIENTS

2 medium zucchinis

¼ cup nutritional yeast

1 large egg, beaten

⅓ cup almond flour or gluten-free all-purpose flour

¼ teaspoon asafoetida (optional)

½ teaspoon salt

DIRECTIONS

1. Preheat the oven to 425°F (220°C). Line a baking sheet with parchment paper.

2. Cut each zucchini in half lengthwise and then each half again lengthwise to make eight long sticks per zucchini. Cut these sticks crosswise to make a total of 16 sticks from each zucchini.

3. In a medium bowl, mix together the nutritional yeast, almond flour, salt, and asafoetida (if using).

4. In a separate bowl, whisk the egg.

5. Dip each zucchini stick first in the beaten egg, allowing excess to drip off, then roll in the nutritional yeast mixture to coat all sides evenly.

6. Arrange the coated zucchini sticks on the prepared baking sheet in a single layer.

7. Bake in the preheated oven for 10 minutes, then flip each fry and continue baking for another 10 minutes, or until they are golden and crispy.

8. For extra crispiness, place the baking sheet under the broiler for 2 to 3 minutes, or until the fries are darker golden and crispy.

PER SERVING (about 1 ½ cup)
Calories: 119; Total fat: 6g; Protein: 8g;
Carbohydrates: 5g; Fiber: 4g

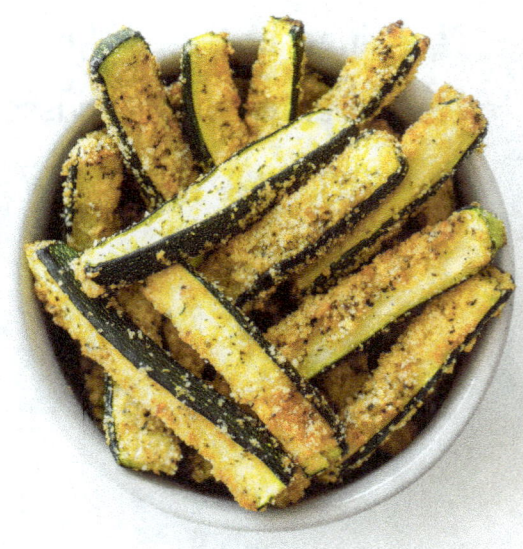

BROCCOLI TOTS

SERVES 3

PREP 20 min

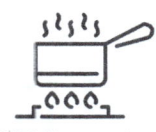
COOK 30 min

READY IN 50 min

INGREDIENTS

2 cups broccoli florets

1 medium potato

1 large egg

3 tablespoons nutritional yeast

¼ cup almond flour (or gluten-free breadcrumbs)

1 teaspoon dried oregano

1 teaspoon dried parsley

½ teaspoon asafoetida (optional)

½ teaspoon salt

DIRECTIONS

1. Preheat the oven to 400°F (200°C) and line a baking sheet with parchment paper.

2. Steam the broccoli florets for about 3-5 minutes, then quickly rinse under cold water to stop the cooking process. Drain well and pat dry with a paper towel.

3. In a food processor, pulse the broccoli until it's finely chopped. You might need to do this in batches. Transfer the chopped broccoli to a clean kitchen towel and squeeze out as much excess water as possible.

4. Meanwhile, place the potato in a saucepan with cold water, ensuring it's completely submerged. Bring to a boil, then reduce the heat to a simmer and cook until the potato is tender, about 12-15 minutes. Allow to cool slightly.

5. Once the potato is cool enough to handle, peel it and grate it using the largest holes on a box grater.

6. In a large mixing bowl, combine the grated potato, chopped broccoli, egg, nutritional yeast, almond flour, oregano, parsley, asafoetida (if using), and salt. Mix well until the ingredients are evenly distributed.

7. Scoop about 1 ½ - 2 tablespoons of the mixture and shape it into a tater-tot form or small cylinders using your hands. Place each tot on the prepared baking sheet.

8. Bake in the preheated oven for 10 minutes, then turn the tots over and continue baking for another 10-15 minutes, or until they are golden brown and crispy.

PER SERVING (about 5 tots) Calories: 153; Total fat: 7g; Protein: 9g; Carbohydrates: 10g; Fiber: 5g

PUMPKIN BREAD

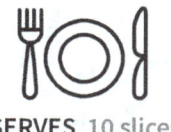
SERVES 10 slices

PREP 10 min

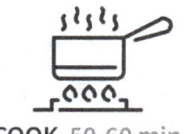
COOK 50-60 min

READY IN 1 hr 10 min

INGREDIENTS

1 cup canned pumpkin purée (not pumpkin pie filling)

2 large eggs

1 ½ cups gluten-free all-purpose flour

¼ teaspoon xanthan gum (omit if your flour blend already includes it)

¼ cup avocado oil or odorless coconut oil

½ cup maple syrup or honey

2 teaspoons vanilla extract

1 teaspoon baking soda

½ teaspoon baking powder

¼ teaspoon salt

1 teaspoon ground cinnamon (omit for healing phase)

DIRECTIONS

1. Preheat the oven to 350°F. Grease a 9 x 5-inch loaf pan with gluten-free cooking spray.

2. In a large bowl, combine the pumpkin, baking soda, baking powder, and salt. Stir in the maple syrup (or honey) and vanilla extract until well mixed. Add the eggs and olive oil to the mixture, blending until smooth.

3. Gradually mix in the gluten-free flour, cinnamon (if using), and xanthan gum until the batter is smooth and thick.

4. Pour the batter into the prepared loaf pan and smooth the top with a spatula. Bake for 50-60 minutes, or until a toothpick inserted into the center comes out clean.

5. Let the bread cool in the pan for about 10 minutes, then turn out onto a wire rack to cool completely.

NOTE

- Store the cooled bread in an airtight container at room temperature. For longer storage, wrap the completely cooled bread in foil or plastic wrap, place in a freezer bag, and freeze for up to 3 months.

PER SERVING (about 1 slice)
Calories: 178; Total fat: 7g; Protein: 2g;
Carbohydrates: 26g; Fiber: 1g

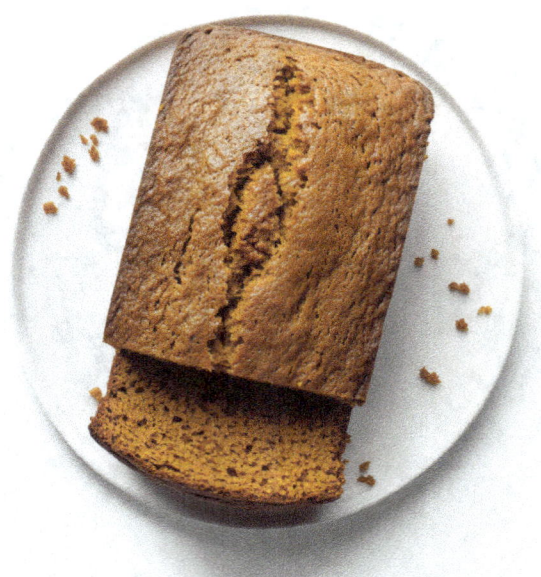

COCONUT COOKIES

 **SERVES** 14-16 cookies

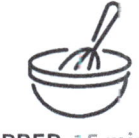 **PREP** 15 min

 **COOK** 12 min

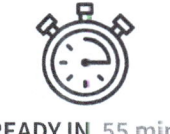 **READY IN** 55 min

INGREDIENTS

1 cup gluten-free all-purpose flour

½ cup oat flour

½ cup unsweetened coconut flakes

1 ripe banana, mashed

1 large egg

1 egg white

2 tablespoons melted coconut oil

¼ cup maple syrup

½ cup pitted dates, chopped (optional)

½ teaspoon baking powder

1 teaspoon vanilla extract

¼ teaspoon salt

DIRECTIONS

1. Preheat the oven to 350°F. Line a large baking sheet with parchment paper.

2. In a medium bowl, combine the mashed banana, coconut oil, maple syrup, egg, egg white, and vanilla extract.

3. In a separate bowl, sift together the gluten-free flour, oat flour, baking powder, and salt.

4. Gradually mix the wet ingredients into the dry ingredients until well combined. Stir in the chopped dates and coconut flakes.

5. Cover the bowl and refrigerate the dough for 30 minutes to firm up.

6. Scoop or roll the dough into 2-tablespoon portions and place them a few inches apart on the prepared baking sheet. Gently press the top of each cookie to flatten slightly.

7. Bake for 9 to 12 minutes, or until the edges are just beginning to turn golden brown.

8. Remove from the oven and let the cookies cool on the baking sheet for a few minutes before transferring them to wire racks to cool completely.

PER SERVING (about 1 cookie) Calories: 103; Total fat: 4g; Protein: 1g; Carbohydrates: 14g; Fiber: 1g

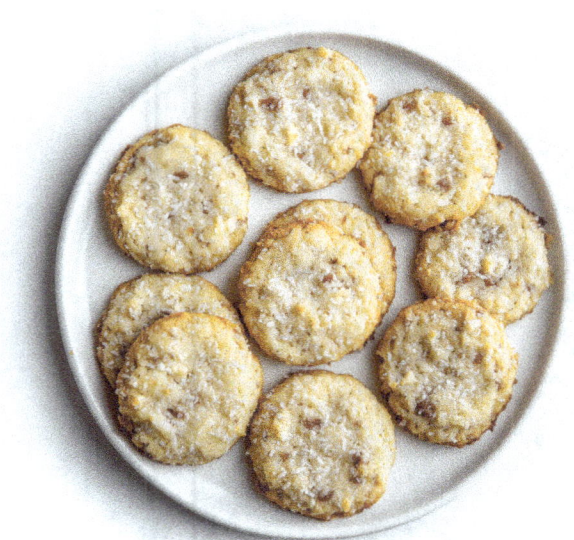

BANANA MUFFINS

 **SERVES** 12 muffins

 **PREP** 15 min

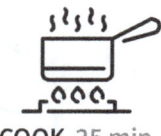 **COOK** 25 min

 **READY IN** 40 min

INGREDIENTS

3 medium ripe bananas, mashed (approximately 1 ½ cups)

1 ¾ cups gluten-free all-purpose flour

¼ cup almond milk or other plant-based milk

¼ cup melted coconut oil

¼ cup maple syrup or honey (adjust based on sweetness of bananas)

1 large egg, beaten

1 teaspoon baking soda

½ teaspoon baking powder

1 teaspoon vanilla extract (optional)

¼ teaspoon salt

DIRECTIONS

1. Preheat the oven to 350°F (177°C). Spray a 12-count muffin pan with nonstick cooking spray or line with cupcake liners.

2. In a medium bowl, whisk together the flour, baking soda, baking powder, and salt. Set aside.

3. In a large bowl, combine the coconut oil and maple syrup or honey. Mix in the egg, mashed bananas, almond milk, and vanilla extract (if using) until well blended.

4. Gradually add the dry ingredients to the wet ingredients, stirring just until combined.

5. Spoon the batter evenly into the prepared muffin pan.

6. Bake for 20-25 minutes, or until a toothpick inserted into the center of a muffin comes out clean.

7. Allow the muffins to cool in the pan for a few minutes before transferring them to a wire rack to cool completely.

PER SERVING (about 1 muffin)
Calories: 152; Total fat: 5g; Protein: 1g; Carbohydrates: 23g; Fiber: 1g

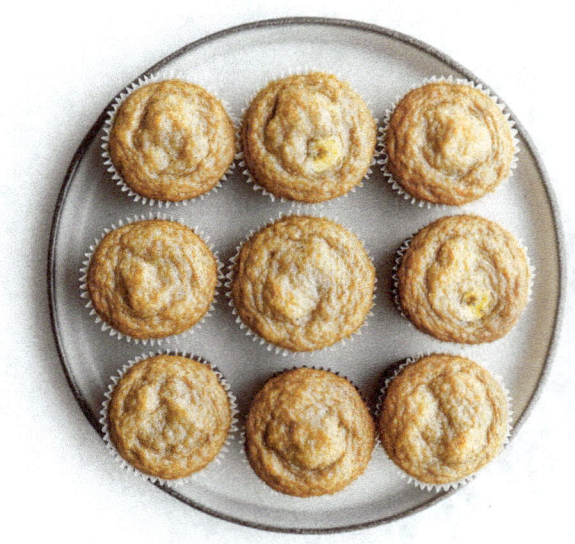

CAROB CAKE

SERVES 8 slices

PREP 10 min

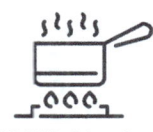
COOK 30 min

READY IN 40 min

INGREDIENTS

- ¾ cup gluten-free all-purpose flour
- 5 tablespoons carob powder
- 2 eggs
- ½ cup maple syrup or honey
- 3 tablespoons melted coconut oil
- ½ teaspoon baking soda
- 1 teaspoon vanilla extract
- ¼ teaspoon salt

DIRECTIONS

1. Preheat the oven to 325°F (163°C) Grease an 8x8-inch baking pan and set aside.

2. In a medium bowl, whisk together the flour, carob powder, baking soda, and salt.

3. In a separate bowl, combine the eggs, maple syrup or honey, coconut oil, and vanilla extract. Whisk until smooth.

4. Gradually add the dry ingredients to the wet ingredients, stirring until just combined.

5. Pour the batter into the prepared baking pan, spreading it evenly.

6. Bake for 25-30 minutes, or until a toothpick inserted into the center of the cake comes out clean.

7. Allow the cake to cool in the pan before cutting into squares.

PER SERVING (about 1 slice) Calories: 160; Total fat: 6g; Protein: 2g; Carbohydrates: 24g; Fiber: 2g

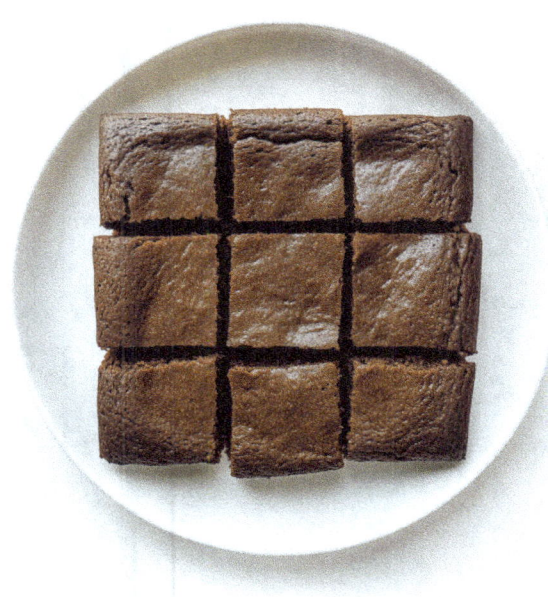

OATMEAL BARS

SERVES 10 bars

PREP 15 min

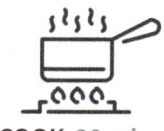

COOK 20 min

READY IN 35 min

INGREDIENTS

2 ½ cups quick-cooking oats

2 large eggs

½ cup unsweetened applesauce (or substitute with mashed banana)

½ cup maple syrup or honey (reduce maple syrup to ¼ cup if using banana)

¾ cup unsweetened almond milk

1 teaspoon vanilla extract

1 ½ teaspoons baking powder

½ teaspoon baking soda

½ teaspoon salt

1 teaspoon ground cinnamon (omit for healing phase)

DIRECTIONS

1. Preheat the oven to 350°F (175°C). Grease a 9x9-inch square baking pan or line it with parchment paper for easy removal.

2. In a large mixing bowl, whisk together eggs, almond milk, applesauce or mashed banana, and vanilla extract until well combined.

3. Add oats, maple syrup or honey, baking powder, baking soda, salt, and cinnamon (if using). Stir together until fully combined.

4. Fold in any optional mix-ins of your choice.

5. Pour the batter into the prepared baking pan, spreading evenly.

6. Bake in the preheated oven for 20-25 minutes, or until the edges are golden brown and a toothpick inserted in the center comes out clean.

7. Allow the bars to cool in the pan for 5-10 minutes before slicing into 16 bars.

PER SERVING (about 1 bar)
Calories: 145; Total fat: 2g; Protein: 4g;
Carbohydrates: 24g; Fiber: 2g

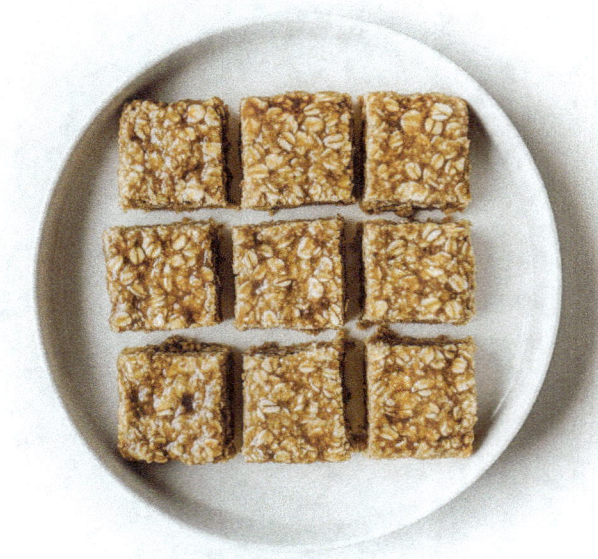

WATERMELON SORBET

SERVES 2

PREP 10 min

COOK n/a

READY IN 12 min

INGREDIENTS

2 cups fresh seedless watermelon, cut into 1-2 inch chunks

⅔ cup unsweetened coconut milk

1 tablespoon maple syrup or honey

1-inch piece of ginger, peeled and grated

DIRECTIONS

1. Freeze the watermelon chunks overnight.

2. Place the frozen watermelon, coconut milk, ginger, and maple syrup in a blender. Pulse about 10 times to combine. Stir with a spoon.

3. Blend on high until smooth, adding more coconut milk if necessary to achieve desired consistency.

4. For a soft texture, serve immediately. For a firmer texture, transfer to a freezer-safe container and freeze for 3-4 hours.

PER SERVING (about 1 cup) Calories: 70; Total fat: 1g; Protein: 1g; Carbohydrates: 14g; Fiber: 1g

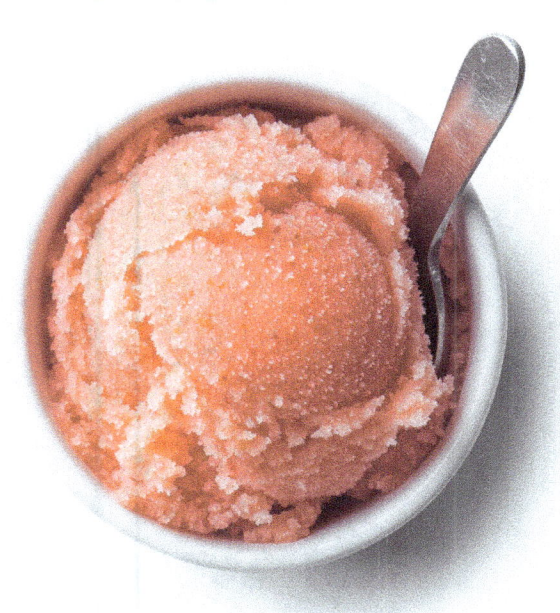

SPIRULINA NICE CREAM

SERVES 2

PREP 10 min

COOK n/a

READY IN 12 min

INGREDIENTS

3 ripe bananas, sliced and frozen

¼ cup almond milk or other plant-based milk

1 teaspoon blue or green spirulina

DIRECTIONS

1. Take the sliced frozen bananas out of the freezer and allow them to thaw for about 5 minutes.

2. Place the bananas, almond milk, and spirulina in a blender.

3. Blend on high until the mixture reaches a soft and creamy consistency. Use a tamper if available to push the ingredients down into the blades for a smoother blend.

4. Serve the nice cream immediately for the best texture or transfer it to a freezer-safe container and freeze if a firmer consistency is desired.

PER SERVING (about 1 cup)
Calories: 168; Total fat: 1g; Protein: 2.6g; Carbohydrates: 37g; Fiber: 4.7g

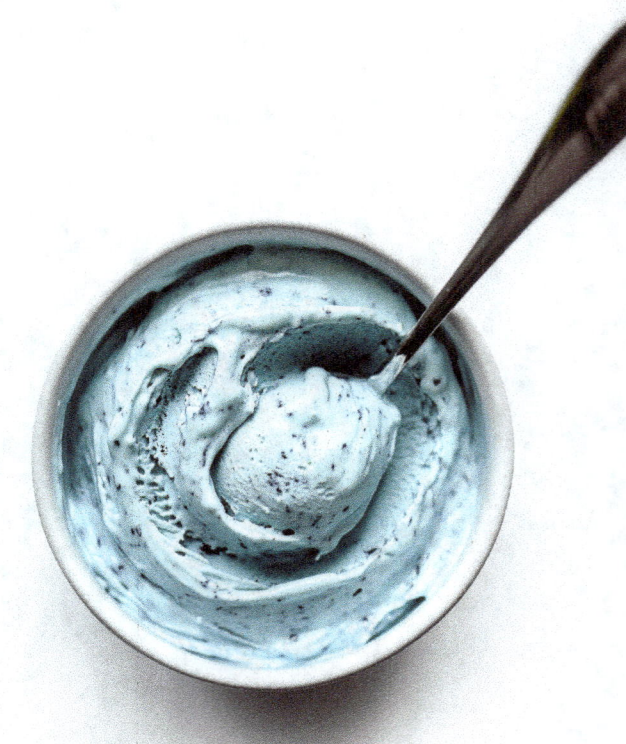

PUMPKIN MUFFINS

SERVES 12 muffins

PREP 10 min

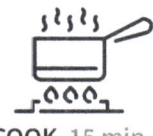

COOK 15 min

READY IN 25 min

INGREDIENTS

1 ¼ cups pumpkin purée

1 ½ cups gluten-free all-purpose flour

2 large eggs

1 teaspoon vanilla extract

¼ cup melted coconut oil

½ cup maple syrup or honey

½ teaspoon baking powder

1 teaspoon baking soda

1 teaspoon ground cinnamon (omit for healing phase)

DIRECTIONS

1. Preheat the oven to 350°F. Generously spray a 12-cup muffin pan with non-stick cooking spray.

2. In a mixing bowl, combine the pumpkin purée, eggs, vanilla extract, and melted coconut oil. Stir until well blended.

3. Add the gluten-free flour, maple syrup (or honey), baking powder, baking soda, and cinnamon (if using). Mix until the batter is smooth.

4. Divide the batter evenly among the 12 muffin cups, filling each nearly to the top.

5. Bake in the preheated oven for 15 to 17 minutes, or until a toothpick inserted into the center of a muffin comes out clean.

6. Remove the muffin pan from the oven and allow the muffins to cool in the pan for about 10 to 15 minutes before transferring them to a wire rack to cool completely.

PER SERVING (1 muffin) Calories: 150; Total fat: 5g; Protein: 2g Carbohydrates: 22g; Fiber: 1g

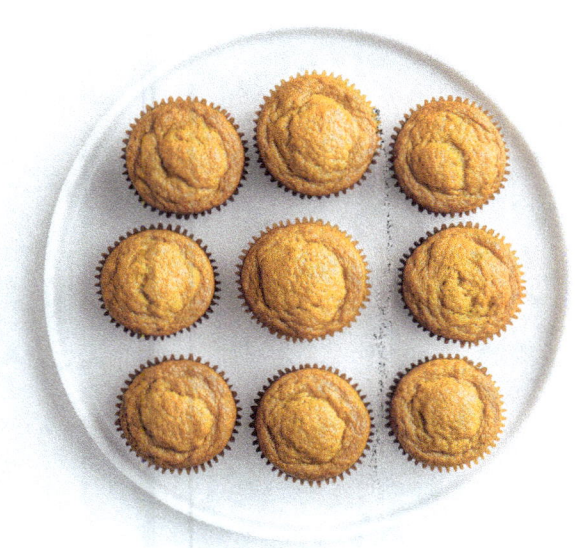

CRISPY CARROT CHIPS

 SERVES 2  PREP 10 min 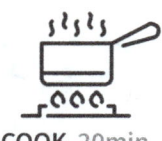 COOK 20min  READY IN 30 min

INGREDIENTS

3 medium carrots

1 tablespoons olive oil or melted coconut oil

¼ tablespoon salt

¼ teaspoon ground cumin

¼ teaspoon ground cinnamon (optional, for maintenance phase)

DIRECTIONS

1. Preheat your oven to 425°F (220°C). Line several large baking sheets with parchment paper.

2. Trim the tops off the carrots. Using a mandolin slicer on the thinnest setting, slice the carrots diagonally starting from the thick end to create elongated, paper-thin slices. Stop slicing when you reach the thinner end of the carrot to avoid waste.

3. In a large mixing bowl, combine the carrot slices, olive oil, sea salt, cumin, and cinnamon (if using). Toss until the slices are evenly coated.

4. Spread the carrot slices in a single layer on the prepared baking sheets, ensuring they do not overlap.

5. Bake in the preheated oven for 12-15 minutes until the edges start to curl up and turn crisp.

6. Flip all the chips and continue baking for an additional 5-8 minutes until the other side is crisp.

7. Allow the chips to cool completely on the baking sheets before transferring them to an airtight container, where they can be stored for up to 2 weeks.

PER SERVING (about 1 cup)
Calories: 97; Total fat: 7g; Protein: 1g;
Carbohydrates: 6g; Fiber: 2g

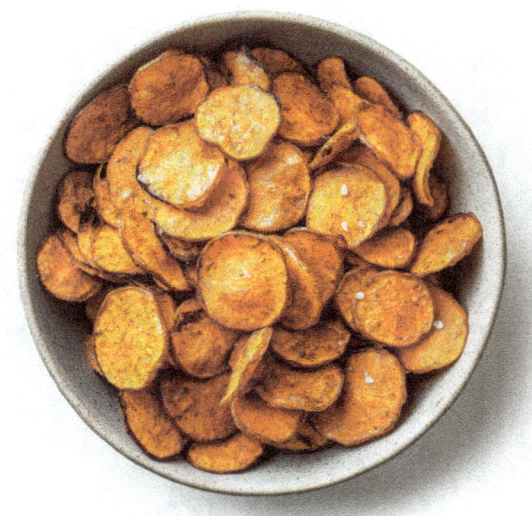

GINGERBREAD COOKIES

 **SERVES** 10-12 cookies

 **PREP** 30 min

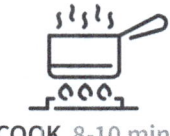 **COOK** 8-10 min

 **READY IN** 1 h 20 min

INGREDIENTS

1 ½ cups almond flour

½ cup coconut flour

2 Medjool dates, pitted

3 tablespoons maple syrup or honey

2 tablespoons avocado oil or odorless coconut oil

½ teaspoon baking soda

2 teaspoons ground ginger

1 teaspoon vanilla extract

½ teaspoon ground cinnamon (optional, for maintenance phase)

¼ teaspoon ground nutmeg (optional, for maintenance phase)

¼ teaspoon salt

DIRECTIONS

1. In a blender, combine the dates, maple syrup (or honey), avocado oil, and 2 tablespoons of water. Blend until smooth, about 1 minute.

2. Add almond flour, coconut flour, baking soda, ginger, vanilla, cinnamon, nutmeg, and salt to the blender. Pulse until a dough forms. Use a spatula to manually mix and scrape down the sides between pulses to ensure even mixing.

3. Transfer the dough to a large mixing bowl. Knead by hand to ensure all ingredients are well combined.

4. Form the dough into a ball, cover the bowl with plastic wrap, and refrigerate for 2 hours to firm up.

5. Preheat your oven to 350°F (175°C). Line two baking sheets with parchment paper.

6. Place the chilled dough between two sheets of parchment paper on a flat surface. Roll out the dough to ¼ inch thickness.

7. Using a gingerbread man cookie cutter, cut out cookies and place them on the prepared baking sheets about 1 inch apart. Re-roll any scraps and repeat until all dough is used.

8. Bake in the preheated oven for 8-10 minutes, or until the edges are slightly browned. Be careful not to overbake as the cookies can burn easily.

9. Allow the cookies to cool on the baking sheets before transferring to a storage container. They can be stored in the refrigerator for up to 2 days.

PER SERVING (about 1 cookie) Calories: 133; Total fat: 9g; Protein: 4g; Carbohydrates: 6g; Fiber: 3g

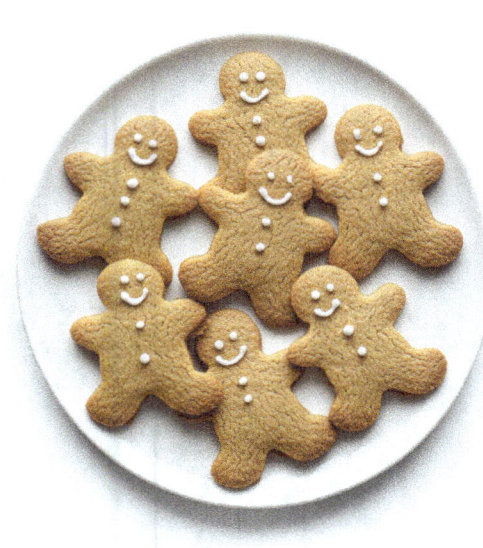

CREAMY CAROB MOUSSE

SERVES 4

PREP 10 min

COOK n/a

READY IN 10 min

INGREDIENTS

2 ripe Hass avocados, peeled and pitted

4 Medjool dates, pitted

¼ cup carob powder

½ cup unsweetened almond milk

2 tablespoons maple syrup or honey

1 teaspoon vanilla extract

Pinch of salt

2 tablespoons shredded coconut, toasted (optional, for garnish)

DIRECTIONS

1. Add the avocados, dates, carob powder, almond milk, maple syrup, vanilla extract, and a pinch of salt to a food processor.

2. Process until the mixture is smooth and creamy, which may take about 3 minutes. Pause to scrape down the sides of the bowl occasionally to ensure all ingredients are well incorporated.

3. Once fully blended to a smooth consistency, taste and adjust the sweetness or saltiness according to your preference.

4. Divide the mousse into two serving bowls. If desired, garnish with toasted shredded coconut.

5. Serve immediately for the best texture or freeze for later use.

PER SERVING (about ½ cup)
Calories: 89; Total fat: 11g; Protein: 2g; Carbohydrates: 27g; Fiber: 8g

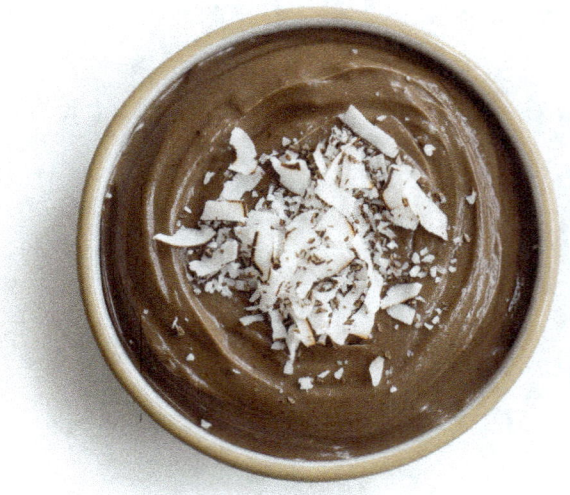

PUMPKIN DONUTS

SERVES 12 donuts

PREP 20 min

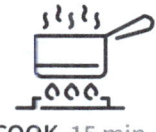
COOK 15 min

READY IN 35 min

INGREDIENTS

1 cup canned pumpkin purée (not pumpkin pie filling)

1 ½ cups all-purpose gluten-free flour

½ teaspoon xanthan gum (omit if your flour includes it)

2 large eggs

1 teaspoon baking powder

½ cup maple syrup or honey

¼ cup avocado oil or odorless coconut oil

1 teaspoon vanilla extract

½ teaspoon ground cinnamon (optional, for maintenance phase)

½ teaspoon salt

DIRECTIONS

1. Preheat the oven to 350°F and grease a 12-cavity donut pan with gluten-free cooking spray.

2. In a large bowl, mix the pumpkin, eggs, oil, maple syrup or honey, and vanilla extract until fully combined.

3. Add the gluten-free flour, xanthan gum (if using), baking powder, salt, and cinnamon. Mix until the batter is thick and smooth.

4. Transfer the batter to a large plastic storage bag or a piping bag. Cut the tip off and pipe the batter evenly into the donut pan.

5. Bake for 14-16 minutes until the donuts are golden brown and set.

6. Transfer to a wire rack or plate to cool.

7. Serve warm or allow to cool completely. Store leftovers in an airtight container, or freeze for up to 3 months for later enjoyment.

PER SERVING (1 donut) Calories: 148; Total Fat: 5g; Protein: 2g
Carbohydrates: 21g; Fiber: 1g

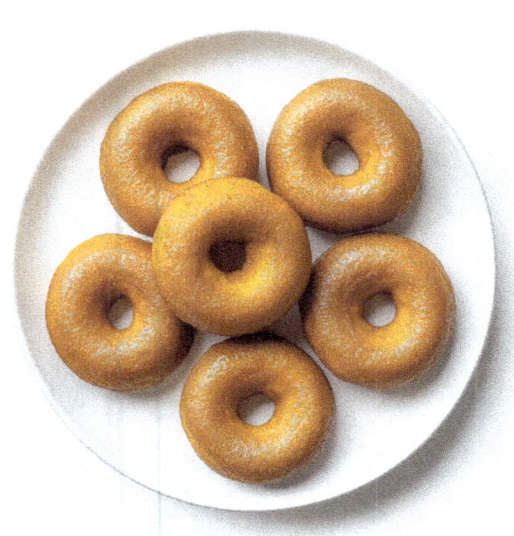

PUFFED RICE BARS

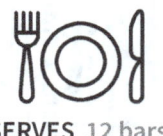 **SERVES** 12 bars

 **PREP** 10 min

 **COOK** n/a

 **READY IN** 40 min

INGREDIENTS

3 cups plain puffed rice cereal

¼ cup nut butter (ensure it's free from added sugars or oils)

⅓ cup maple syrup

¼ cup water

1 tablespoon carob powder (optional, for a chocolatey flavor)

DIRECTIONS

1. In a small saucepan, combine the nut butter, maple syrup, water, and carob powder (if using). Heat the mixture over medium heat, stirring continuously until it becomes smooth and well combined.

2. Place the puffed rice cereal in a large mixing bowl.

3. Pour the warm nut butter mixture over the puffed rice cereal. Stir well until all the cereal is evenly coated.

4. Line a baking sheet with parchment paper. Spoon the cereal mixture onto the lined baking sheet, spreading it out evenly.

5. Place the baking sheet in the freezer for about 30 minutes to allow the bars to set.

6. After the bars have set, remove them from the freezer and cut them into desired sizes.

7. Store the puffed rice bars in the refrigerator in an airtight container.

PER SERVING (1 bar) Calories: 70; Total fat: 3g; Protein: 1g; Carbohydrates: 9g; Fiber: 1g

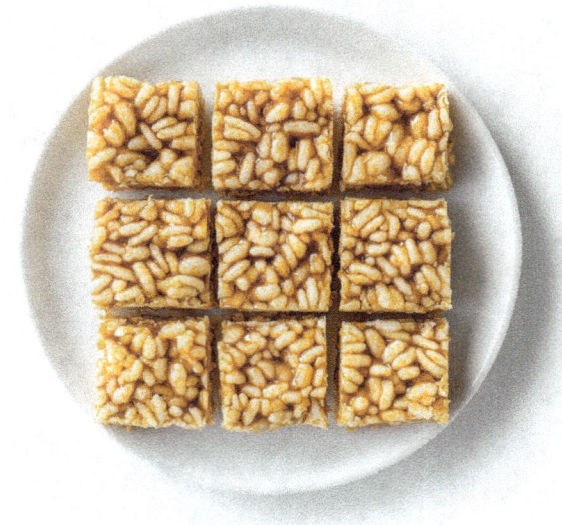

SWEET POTATO BROWNIES

SERVES 16 pieces

PREP 10 min

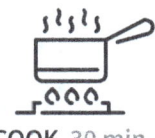
COOK 30 min

READY IN 40 min

INGREDIENTS

1 ½ cups mashed sweet potatoes (roast, boil, or steam beforehand)

⅓ cup carob powder

¼ cup oat flour or almond flour

¼ cup nut butter of choice or melted coconut oil (see note)

¼ cup maple syrup or honey

1 teaspoon vanilla extract (optional)

Pinch of salt

DIRECTIONS

1. Set your oven to 350°F (175°C). Grease an 8x8-inch baking pan and line it with parchment paper. Set aside.

2. Add all ingredients to a food processor and blend until smooth. Alternatively, combine all the ingredients in a mixing bowl, starting with the wet ingredients followed by the dry ingredients to ensure even mixing.

3. Pour the batter into your prepared pan. Use a spatula to spread the batter evenly across the pan, smoothing out the top.

4. Place the pan in the preheated oven and bake for 25-30 minutes, or until the center feels firm to the touch and the edges start to pull away from the sides of the pan.

5. Allow the brownies to cool in the pan completely before slicing. This will help them set properly, making them easier to cut into squares. Serve warm or at room temperature.

NOTES

- If choosing nut butter, ensure it's smooth and doesn't contain added sugar or oils.

- The choice between oat flour and almond flour can affect the texture; oat flour tends to make them slightly denser than almond flour.

PER SERVING (about 1 piece) Calories: 77; Total fat: 3g; Protein: 2g; Carbohydrates: 10g; Fiber: 2g

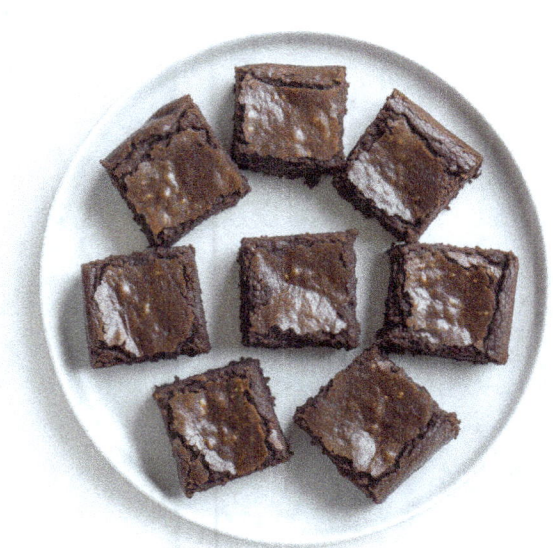

DATE ENERGY BALLS

 **SERVES** 12-14 balls

 **PREP** 15 min

 **COOK** n/a

 **READY IN** 15 min

INGREDIENTS

1 cup Medjool dates, pitted

½ cup walnuts (substitute with other nuts if preferred)

½ cup unsweetened shredded coconut

½ teaspoon vanilla extract (optional)

¼ teaspoon salt

DIRECTIONS

1. Place the pitted dates, walnuts, shredded coconut, vanilla extract (if using), and salt in a food processor fitted with an "S" blade.

2. Pulse the mixture until it becomes crumbly but sticks together when pressed between your fingers. Do not over-process.

3. Using a 1-ounce cookie scoop or a tablespoon, scoop the mixture and press it together firmly.

4. Roll between your hands to form balls, ensuring each one is compact.

5. The date energy balls can be enjoyed immediately or stored for later.

6. Place them in an airtight container and refrigerate for up to 2 weeks or freeze for up to 3 months.

NOTE

- If the mixture feels too dry to form into balls, you can add a little more dates or a teaspoon of water to help it bind.

PER SERVING (1 ball) Calories: 96; Total fat: 4g; Protein: 1g; Carbohydrates: 13g; Fiber: 2g

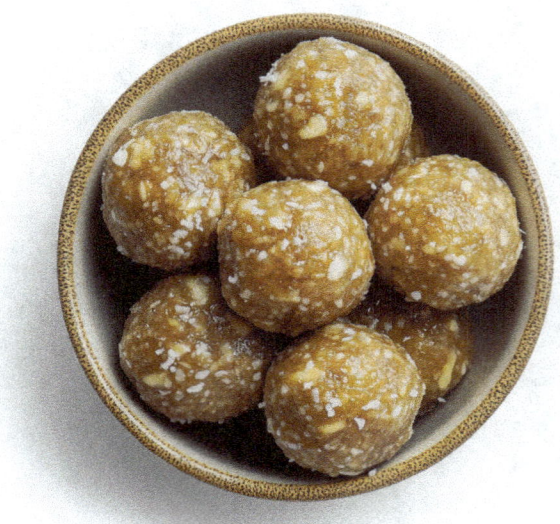

BAKED YUCA FRIES

SERVES 4

PREP 20 min

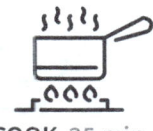

COOK 25 min

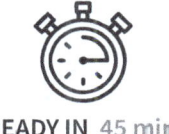

READY IN 45 min

INGREDIENTS

2 large yucas

2 tablespoons olive oil

¾ teaspoon salt

Avocado Sauce:

1 ripe avocado

2 tablespoons almond milk (or ¼ cup plain dairy-free yogurt for maintenance phase)

Zest from 1 lemon

¼ cup fresh cilantro

Salt to taste

DIRECTIONS

1. Preheat the oven to 450°F.

2. Bring a large pot of water to a boil. Trim the ends off each yuca, cut them in half crosswise, and stand them on their cut ends. Carefully cut away the waxy outer peel with a sharp knife.

3. Slice each yuca half lengthwise, then slice again to make quarters, resulting in 16 pieces total. Remove the fibrous core from each piece.

4. Boil the yuca pieces until fork-tender, about 8-10 minutes. Remove with a slotted spoon and transfer to a paper towel-lined cutting board to dry.

5. Pat the yuca dry with additional paper towels, then transfer to a large mixing bowl. Toss with olive oil and salt until well coated.

6. Spread the yuca on a large baking sheet in a single layer.

7. Bake in the preheated oven for about 25 minutes, or until golden and crispy, flipping halfway through.

8. While the yuca bakes, blend the avocado, almond milk, lemon zest, and cilantro in a blender or food processor until smooth. Season with salt to taste.

9. Serve the baked yuca fries warm with the avocado dipping sauce on the side.

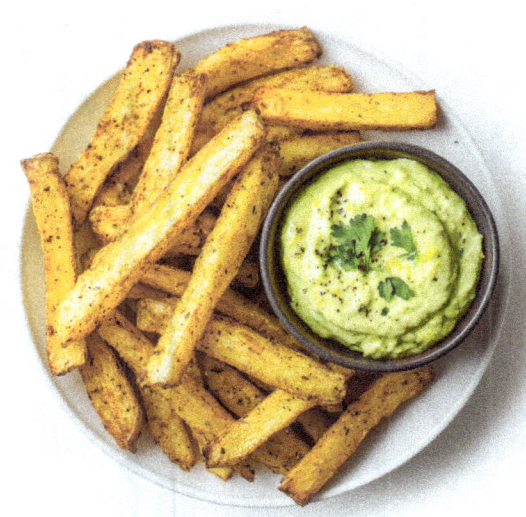

PER SERVING (¼ of the yuca fries) Calories: 298; Total fat: 7g; Protein: 2g; Carbohydrates: 54g; Fiber: 2g

MANGO PUDDING

 **SERVES** 2    **PREP** 10 min    **COOK** 5 min    **READY IN** 2 h 15 min

INGREDIENTS

2 medium mangoes, peeled and chopped

1 cup lite coconut milk or unsweetened almond milk

2-4 tablespoons maple syrup (adjust depending on the sweetness of the mangoes)

½ cup water

1 tablespoon unflavored gelatin

Pinch of salt

DIRECTIONS

1. In a food processor, puree the mango chunks until silky smooth.

2. Add half a cup of the coconut milk and the maple syrup to the pureed mango. Process again until well incorporated.

3. In a small pot, combine the water and the remaining half cup of coconut milk. Heat until it just begins to simmer and is steaming. Remove from heat.

4. Sprinkle the gelatin evenly over the surface and whisk briskly until the gelatin is completely dissolved and no clumps remain.

5. Add the gelatin mixture to the mango puree in the food processor. Process until well incorporated and smooth. Taste and adjust for sweetness if necessary.

6. Pour the mixture into small ramekins or jars. Cover and chill in the fridge until set, at least 2-3 hours. The pudding can be stored in the fridge for 2-3 days.

NOTE

• Using unsweetened almond milk will make the pudding low-fat and slightly less creamy compared to using coconut milk.

PER SERVING (about 1 cup)
Calories: 346; Total fat: 8g; Protein: 5g; Carbohydrates: 64g; Fiber: 3g

CAROB STUFFED DATES

SERVES 10

PREP 15 min

COOK n/a

READY IN 45 min

INGREDIENTS

10 Medjool dates

¼ cup almond butter or peanut butter (no added sugar or oils)

¼ cup chopped or crushed almonds

⅓ cup coconut oil

¼ cup carob powder

2 tablespoons maple syrup

DIRECTIONS

1. Prepare a baking sheet or plate by lining it with parchment paper.

2. Carefully slit each date and remove the pit; arrange them on the prepared parchment paper.

3. In a small bowl, combine the almond butter with 2 tablespoons of the crushed almonds. Mix until well incorporated.

4. Stuff about ½ teaspoon of the almond butter mixture into each date.

5. Melt the coconut oil in a saucepan over low heat or in the microwave for about 30-60 seconds.

6. Once melted, remove the coconut oil from heat. Gradually whisk in the carob powder until smooth, ensuring there are no lumps. Stir the maple syrup into the carob mixture until well combined.

7. Dip each stuffed date into the carob mixture using a fork, ensuring they are completely coated.

8. Transfer the coated dates back to the parchment paper and sprinkle with the remaining crushed almonds.

9. Refrigerate the dates until the carob coating is set, about 30 minutes.

10. Store the carob stuffed dates in a sealed container in the refrigerator for up to a week.

PER SERVING (1 stufed date) Calories: 214; Total fat: 12g; Protein: 2g; Carbohydrates: 23g; Fiber: 3g

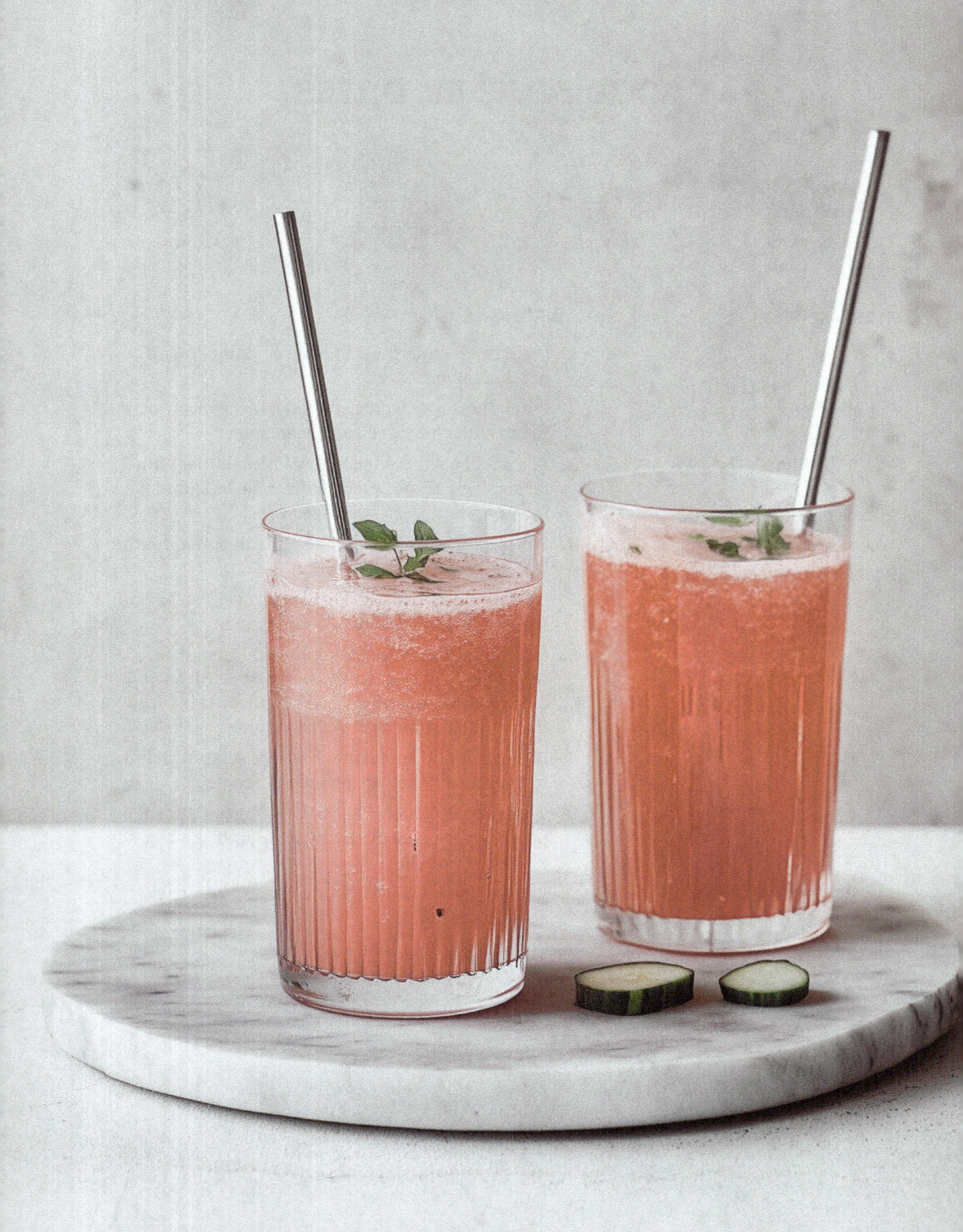

CHAPTER EIGHT

SMOOTHIES & DRINKS

BANANA MANGO SMOOTHIE

 **SERVES** 1

 **PREP** 5 min

 **COOK** n/a

 **READY IN** 7 min

INGREDIENTS

1 medium banana, sliced

¼ cup fresh or frozen mango

½ teaspoon fresh ginger, grated

½ cup almond milk or other plant-based milk

DIRECTIONS

1. Place the banana, mango, ginger, and almond milk in a blender.

2. Blend on high until the mixture is completely smooth. Adjust the consistency by adding a bit more almond milk if needed.

3. Pour the smoothie into a glass and serve immediately for the freshest taste.

PER SERVING (about 1 cup)
Calories: 158; Total fat: 1g; Protein: 2g;
Carbohydrates: 33g; Fiber: 4g

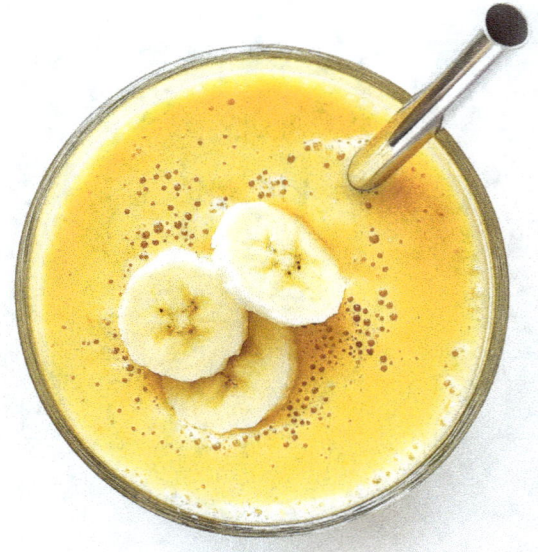

STRAWBERRY BEET SMOOTHIE

SERVES 2

PREP 5 min

COOK n/a

READY IN 7 min

INGREDIENTS

1 cup cooked beets, chopped

1 cup unsweetened almond milk

½ cup frozen strawberries

1 tablespoon maple syrup or honey

DIRECTIONS

1. Place the cooked beets, almond milk, frozen strawberries, and maple syrup (or honey) in a blender.

2. Blend until smooth and creamy.

3. Pour the smoothie into glasses and serve immediately.

NOTE

• It's advisable to cook the beets before using them, as raw vegetables may cause stomach issues during the healing phase.

PER SERVING (about 1 ¼ cups) Calories: 89; Total fat: 1g; Protein: 2g; Carbohydrates: 17g; Fiber: 2.6g

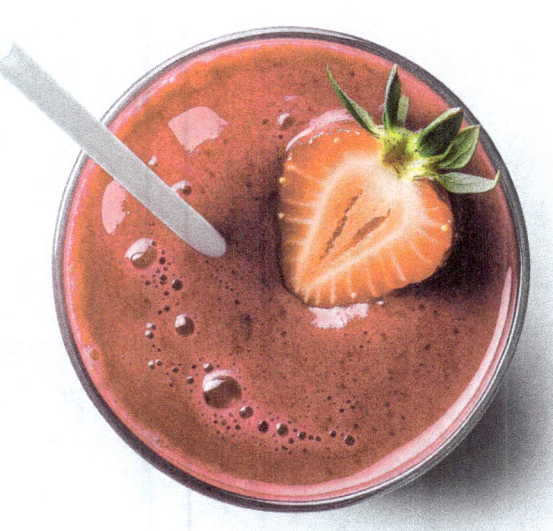

WATERMELON CUCUMBER JUICE

SERVES 1

PREP 5 min

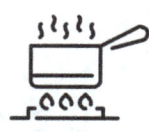

COOK n/a

READY IN 5 min

INGREDIENTS

1 ½ cups seedless watermelon, cubed

½ cup English cucumber, sliced

1 teaspoon chia seeds (omit for healing phase)

½ teaspoon lemon zest (optional)

DIRECTIONS

1. Add the cubed watermelon, sliced cucumber, and lemon zest (if using) to a blender. Blend until smooth.

2. Strain the juice through a fine mesh sieve or cheesecloth to remove any pulp for a smoother consistency.

3. Stir the chia seeds into the strained juice.

4. Refrigerate the juice for at least 20 minutes to allow the chia seeds to swell and thicken the juice slightly.

5. Serve chilled for a refreshing drink.

PER SERVING (about 2 cups)
Calories: 66; Total fat: 1g; Protein: 1g;
Carbohydrates: 11g; Fiber: 2g

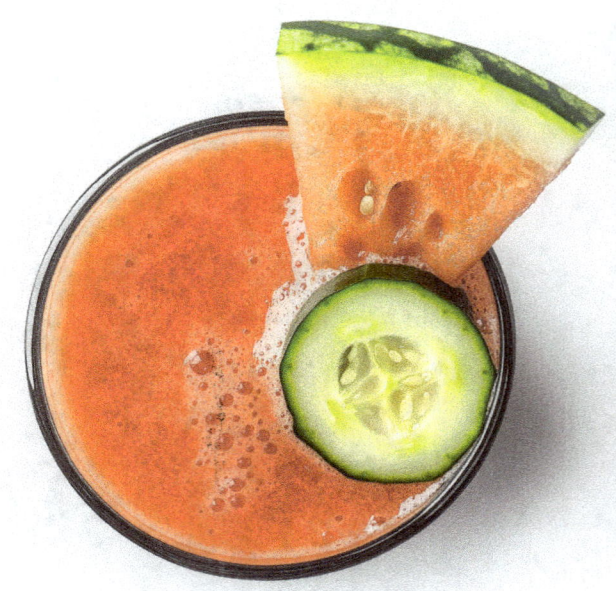

MELON SMOOTHIE

SERVES 2

PREP 5 min

COOK n/a

READY IN 7 min

INGREDIENTS

1 ½ cups cantaloupe, chopped (alternative melons can be used)

1 ½ cups almond milk or other plant-based milk

½ cup plain non-dairy yogurt (optional, for maintenance phase)

1-2 tablespoons maple syrup or honey

DIRECTIONS

1. Place the chopped cantaloupe, almond milk, non-dairy yogurt (if using), and maple syrup into a blender.

2. Blend all ingredients until smooth.

3. Pour the smoothie into glasses and serve immediately for a refreshing drink.

PER SERVING (about 1 ½ cups) Calories: 93 Total fat: 2g; Protein: 2g; Carbohydrates: 15g; Fiber: 1g

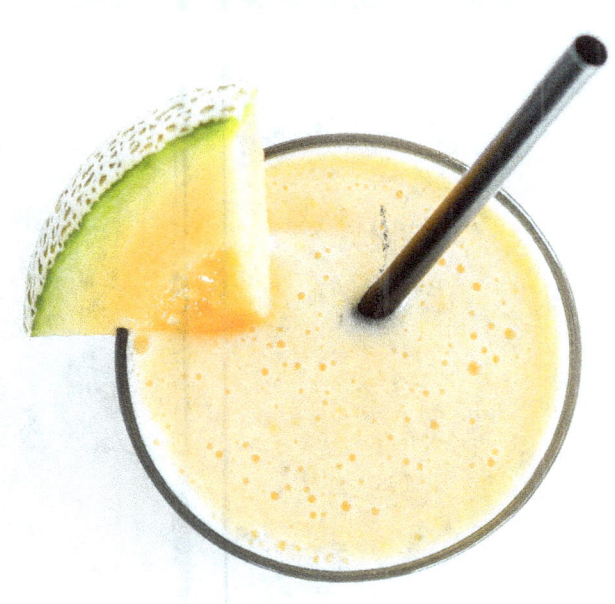

CAROB BANANA SMOOTHIE

SERVES 1

PREP 5 min

COOK n/a

READY IN 7 min

INGREDIENTS

1 frozen banana

½ cup almond milk or other plant-based milk

1 tablespoon carob powder

1 tablespoon almond butter

1 tablespoon maple syrup or honey (optional)

DIRECTIONS

1. Combine the frozen banana, almond milk, carob powder, almond butter, and maple syrup (if using) in a blender.

2. Blend until smooth. For a thinner smoothie, add additional milk until you achieve your desired consistency.

3. Pour the smoothie into a glass and serve immediately for a delicious and energizing treat.

PER SERVING (about 1 cup)
Calories: 233; Total fat: 10g; Protein: 5g;
Carbohydrates: 28g; Fiber: 7g

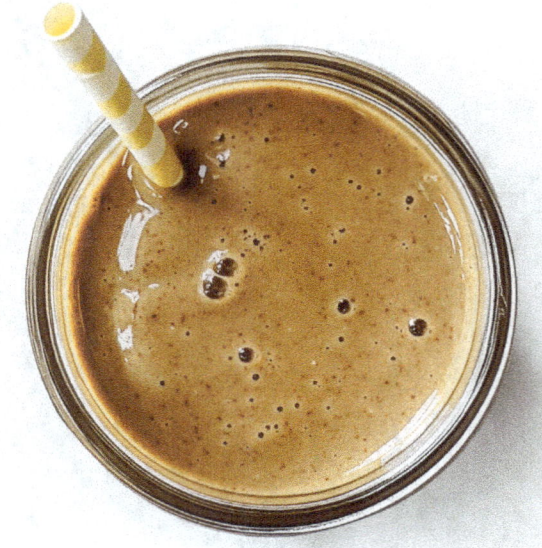

CHAMOMILE LATTE

SERVES 2

PREP 5 min

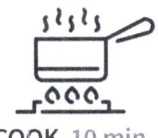
COOK 10 min

READY IN 15 min

INGREDIENTS

1 ½ cups water

1 ½ cups almond milk or other plant-based milk

2 chamomile tea bags (or 2 teaspoons loose leaf tea)

2-4 cloves, crushed

1 cinnamon stick

1 tablespoon maple syrup or honey

DIRECTIONS

1. In a small saucepan, bring the water to a simmer. Add the chamomile tea, cinnamon stick, and cloves. Remove from heat, cover, and allow to steep for 10 minutes.

2. While the tea is steeping, heat the almond milk in another saucepan over medium heat. Whisk constantly until the milk is warm and frothy, about 5 minutes.

3. Remove the tea bags, cinnamon stick, and cloves from the tea. You can strain the mixture to ensure no remnants remain.

4. Stir the maple syrup or honey into the tea mixture.

5. Pour the warm frothy milk into the tea and stir gently to combine.

6. Serve the latte immediately, enjoying the soothing flavors of chamomile enhanced with spices.

PER SERVING (about 1 cup) Calories: 52; Total fat: 2g; Protein: 0g; Carbohydrates: 7g; Fiber: 0g

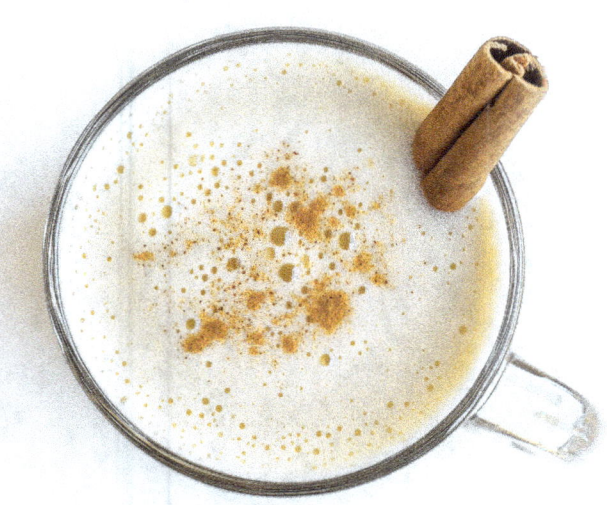

APPLE CARROT BEET JUICE

 SERVES 1

 PREP 10 min

 COOK n/a

 READY IN 10 min

INGREDIENTS

1 Red Delicious apple, peeled, cored, and quartered

1 small beet, cut into chunks

1-2 medium carrots, peeled and ends trimmed

½ teaspoon fresh ginger, peeled

½ cup water

DIRECTIONS

1. Place the apple, beet, carrots, ginger, and water in a blender. Blend on high speed until everything is completely smooth, about 1-2 minutes. Use a tamper if necessary to ensure even blending.

2. Set a fine mesh strainer over a large bowl and pour the blended mixture through it. Use a spoon or spatula to press down on the pulp to extract as much juice as possible.

3. Discard the pulp. Transfer the strained juice into a serving glass. You can enjoy it immediately or refrigerate it to chill before drinking.

PER SERVING (about 1 cup)
Calories: 185; Total fat: 0g; Protein: 2g; Carbohydrates: 34g; Fiber: 9g

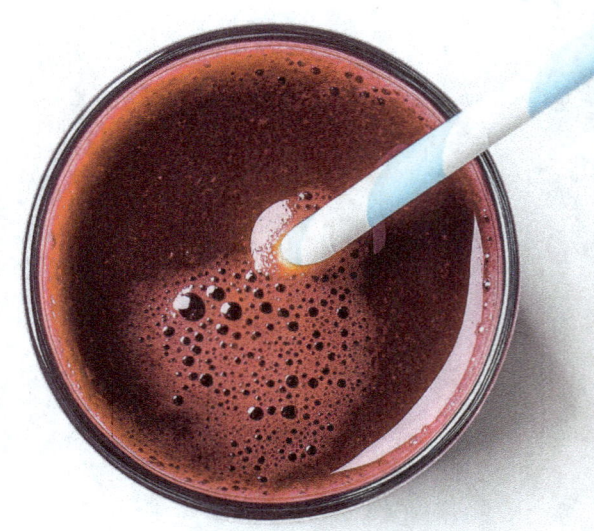

PEAR GINGER SMOOTHIE

 **SERVES** 2

 **PREP** 5 min

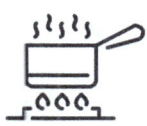 **COOK** n/a

 **READY IN** 7 min

INGREDIENTS

2 ripe Bosc pears, peeled and cut into chunks

1 cup almond milk or other plant-based milk

½ cup plain non-dairy yogurt (optional, for maintenance phase; see note)

½ teaspoon fresh ginger, grated

DIRECTIONS

1. Add the pears, almond milk, non-dairy yogurt (if using), and grated ginger to a blender.

2. Blend until smooth.

3. Serve immediately and enjoy the refreshing taste!

NOTE

- If not using non-dairy yogurt, you can add one banana to the blend to achieve a creamy texture.

PER SERVING (about 1 cup) Calories: 190; Total fat: 2g; Protein: 2g; Carbohydrates: 35g; Fiber: 7g

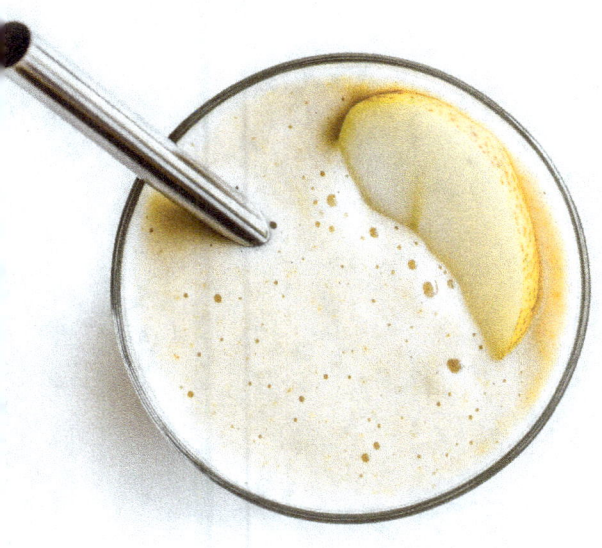

CHICORY LATTE

SERVES 1

PREP 10 min

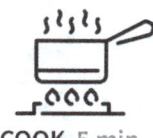
COOK 5 min

READY IN 15 min

INGREDIENTS

1 teaspoon chicory root powder

1 cup water

¼ cup coconut milk or other plant-based milk

1 teaspoon coconut oil

1 teaspoon unflavored gelatin

1 teaspoon maple syrup or honey

½ teaspoon carob powder (optional)

DIRECTIONS

1. Start by brewing your chicory. If using a coffee maker, simply pour the water through the machine with the chicory root powder. Alternatively, bring water to a boil in a small pot, add the chicory root powder, and let it steep for 7-10 minutes before straining.

2. Transfer the brewed chicory to a blender. Add coconut milk, coconut oil, maple syrup or honey, gelatin, and carob powder, if using.

3. Blend on high speed for about one minute or until the mixture becomes frothy.

4. Serve the latte warm and enjoy!

PER SERVING (about 1 cup)
Calories: 87; Total fat: 5g; Protein: 3g;
Carbohydrates: 5g; Fiber: 0g

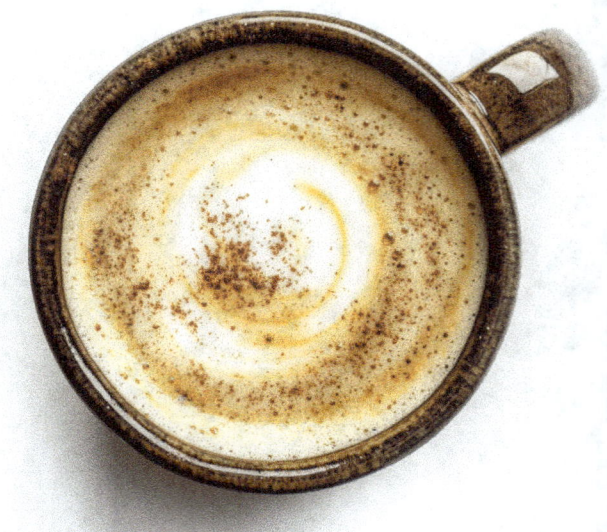

CARDAMON CHAI

 **SERVES** 2

 **PREP** 5 min

 **COOK** 15 min

 **READY IN** 20 min

INGREDIENTS

1 cup almond milk or other plant-based milk

2 cups water

1 ½-inch piece fresh ginger, peeled and thinly sliced

2 star anises

⅛ teaspoon ground cardamom

¼ teaspoon cinnamon powder

¼ teaspoon ground nutmeg

4 dandelion tea bags

1-2 tablespoons maple syrup or honey (adjust sweetness to taste)

DIRECTIONS

1. In a medium-sized saucepan, combine water and almond milk. Bring to a gentle boil over medium heat.

2. Add the sliced ginger, star anises, cardamom, cinnamon, and nutmeg to the boiling liquid. Cover the saucepan, reduce the heat to low, and let simmer for 5–10 minutes to allow the spices to infuse their flavors.

3. Remove from heat. Add the dandelion tea bags, cover, and let steep for an additional 5 minutes.

4. Remove the tea bags and strain the chai through a fine mesh sieve to remove all solids and spices.

5. Stir in maple syrup or honey to sweeten the chai to your liking.

6. Serve the chai warm, enjoying the aromatic blend of spices and the soothing properties of dandelion tea.

PER SERVING (about 1 ½ cups) Calories: 44; Total fat: 1g; Protein: 0g; Carbohydrates: 7g; Fiber: 0g

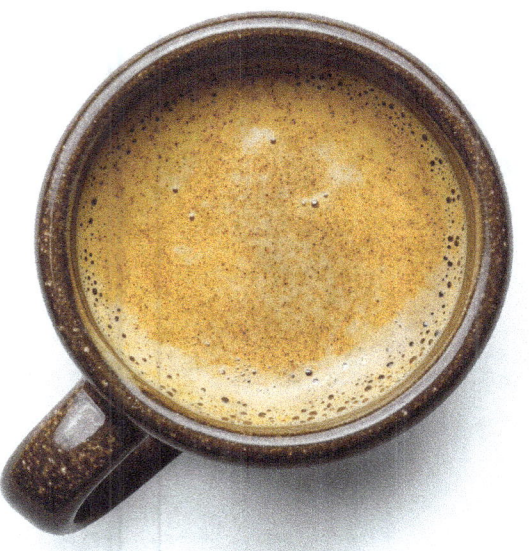

PAPAYA ALOE VERA SMOOTHIE

SERVES 1

PREP 5 min

COOK n/a

READY IN 7 min

INGREDIENTS

1 cup frozen papaya, cubed

1 cup unsweetened almond milk

2-4 ounces aloe vera gel

1 tablespoon maple syrup or honey (adjust sweetness to taste)

DIRECTIONS

1. In a blender, combine the frozen papaya, almond milk, aloe vera gel, and maple syrup or honey.

2. Blend on high until the mixture is smooth and creamy.

3. Pour the smoothie into a large glass and enjoy immediately for the best flavor and nutrient retention.

PER SERVING (about 2 cups)
Calories: 150; Total fat: 3g; Protein: 2g;
Carbohydrates: 27g; Fiber: 2g

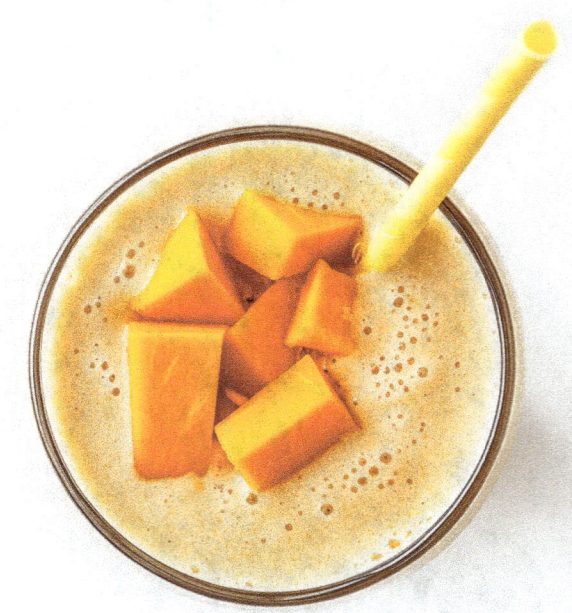

JASMINE MILK TEA

 SERVES 1

 PREP 5 min

 COOK n/a

 READY IN 15 min

INGREDIENTS

2 teaspoons loose jasmine tea leaves (or 2 jasmine tea bags; see note).

¾ cup hot water

½ cup unsweetened almond milk (or other plant-based milk of your choice)

½ cup tapioca pearls (boba), boiled according to package instructions

1 tablespoon maple syrup or honey

DIRECTIONS

1. Pour hot water over the jasmine tea bags or leaves and allow to steep for 3 to 7 minutes, depending on how strong you like your tea. If using loose leaves, strain out the jasmine flowers afterward.

2. Remove the tea bags or strain the tea leaves and stir in the maple syrup or honey until fully dissolved.

3. Mix the almond milk into the sweetened tea, combining well.

4. While the tea is steeping, prepare the tapioca pearls according to the instructions on the package.

5. Place the cooked boba at the bottom of a clear glass. Pour the milky jasmine tea mixture over the boba.

6. You can enjoy the tea warm or chilled. If serving cold, add crushed ice and sip with a wide boba straw.

NOTE

- If using jasmine tea bags that contain green tea, make sure they are decaffeinated.

PER SERVING (about 1 ½ cups) Calories: 342; Total fat: 1g; Protein: 1g; Carbohydrates: 80g; Fiber: 1g

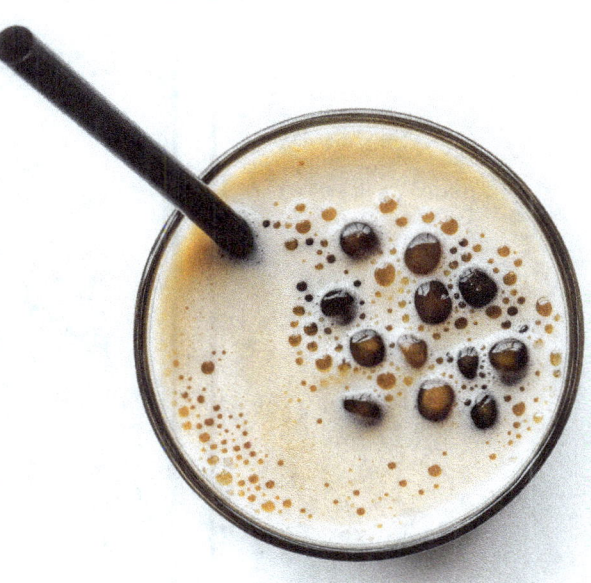

HOT CAROB

 **SERVES** 1

 **PREP** 5 min

 **COOK** 5-10 min

 **READY IN** 10-15 min

INGREDIENTS

1 cup unsweetened almond milk, plus more if needed

1 tablespoon carob powder

1 tablespoon maple syrup or honey

1 tablespoon arrowroot flour (optional, for thickening)

½ teaspoon vanilla extract

A pinch of salt

Dash of cinnamon powder (optional, omit for healing phase)

DIRECTIONS

1. In a saucepan, combine the almond milk, carob powder, honey or maple syrup, and salt. Heat the mixture over medium heat until it begins to steam.

2. If using arrowroot flour for thickening, mix it with a tablespoon of almond milk in a small bowl until smooth to create a slurry.

3. Gradually whisk the arrowroot slurry into the heating carob mixture. Continue stirring until the mixture thickens.

4. Once thickened, remove the saucepan from the heat. Stir in the vanilla extract and a dash of cinnamon if using.

5. Serve the hot carob warm and enjoy immediately.

PER SERVING (about 1 cup)
Calories: 130; Total fat: 3g; Protein: 1g;
Carbohydrates: 24g; Fiber: 2g

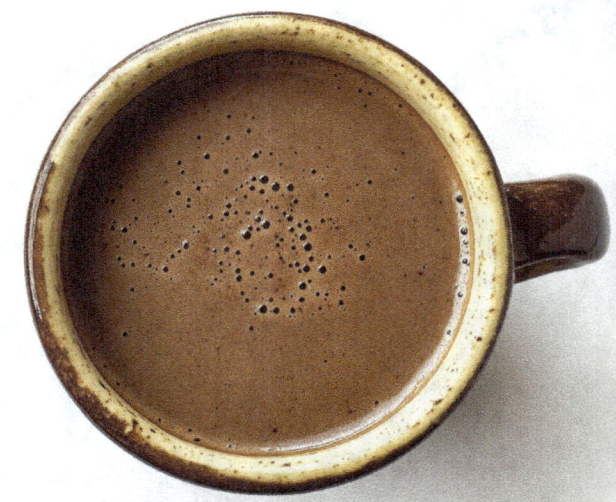

PUMPKIN SMOOTHIE

SERVES 1

PREP 5 min

COOK n/a

READY IN 7 min

INGREDIENTS

½ cup pumpkin purée (ensure it's not pumpkin pie filling)

4 Medjool dates, pitted

1 cup unsweetened almond milk (plus more as needed to adjust consistency)

¼ teaspoon cinnamon powder (optional, for maintenance phase)

DIRECTIONS

1. If the dates are not soft, you may soak them in warm water for about 10 minutes to soften them before blending, which ensures a smoother consistency.

2. Place the pumpkin purée, softened Medjool dates almond milk, and cinnamon (if using) into a blender.

3. Blend on high speed until all ingredients are well combined and the mixture is smooth. If the smoothie is too thick for your liking, gradually add more almond milk until you achieve the desired consistency.

4. Pour the smoothie into glasses and serve immediately.

PER SERVING (about 1 ½ cups) Calories: 347; Total fat: 3g; Protein: 4g; Carbohydrates: 73g; Fiber: 9g

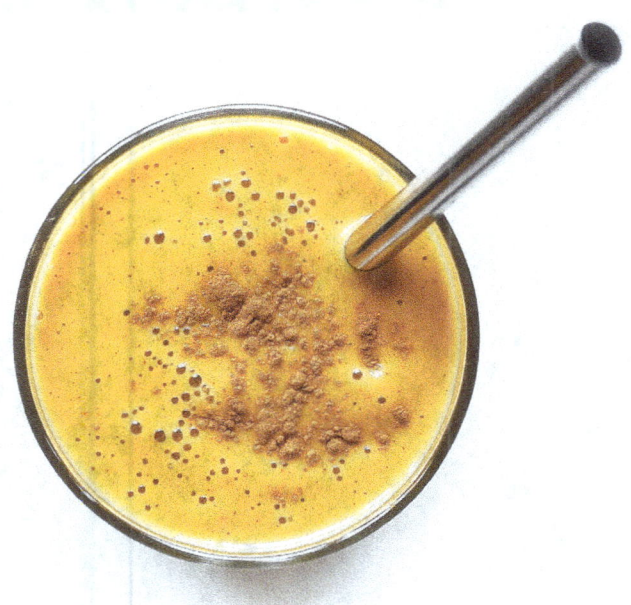

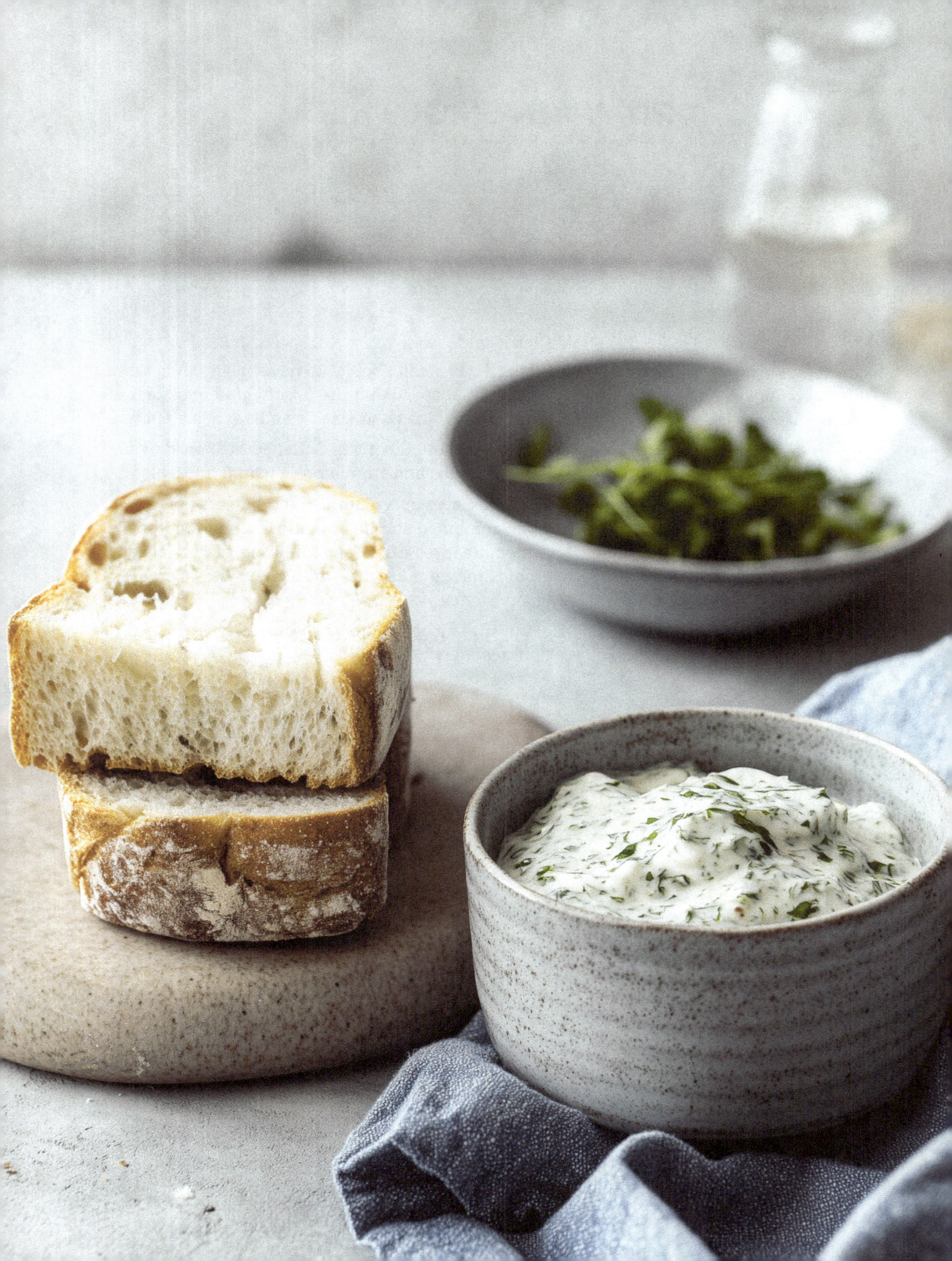

CHAPTER NINE

STAPLES, DRESSINGS, & SAUCES

GLUTEN-FREE BREAD

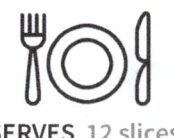
SERVES 12 slices

PREP 15 min

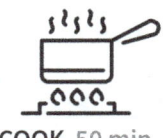
COOK 50 min

READY IN 1 h 15 min

INGREDIENTS

2 ½ cups gluten-free all-purpose flour

2 teaspoons xanthan gum (omit if your flour blend includes it)

1 teaspoon baking powder

1 packet instant yeast (about 2 ¼ teaspoons)

3 tablespoons olive oil or avocado oil

¼ cup maple syrup or honey

1 ½ cups warm water (100-110°F)

3 egg whites

1 teaspoon salt

DIRECTIONS

1. Grease a 9-inch x 5-inch bread pan or a 9-inch x 4-inch Pullman loaf pan. Preheat the oven to 350°F, positioning the rack in the middle.

2. In a large bowl, combine gluten-free flour, xanthan gum (if needed), baking powder, and instant yeast.

3. To the dry mixture, add olive oil, maple syrup, and warm water. Mix with a paddle attachment on low for 1 minute.

4. Add egg whites and salt, mixing on medium for another minute until the batter resembles thick cake batter.

5. Pour the batter into the prepared pan. Cover with greased plastic wrap and a kitchen towel. Let it rise in a warm place for 30 minutes.

6. Bake for 50 minutes or until golden brown and the internal temperature reaches 205-210°F.

7. Allow to cool in the pan for 10 minutes, then transfer to a cooling rack to cool completely to avoid sogginess.

8. Keep in an airtight container at room temperature. Do not slice until ready to serve to maintain freshness.

PER SERVING (1 slice) Calories: 143; Total fat: 4g; Protein: 2g; Carbohydrates: 24g; Fiber: 1g

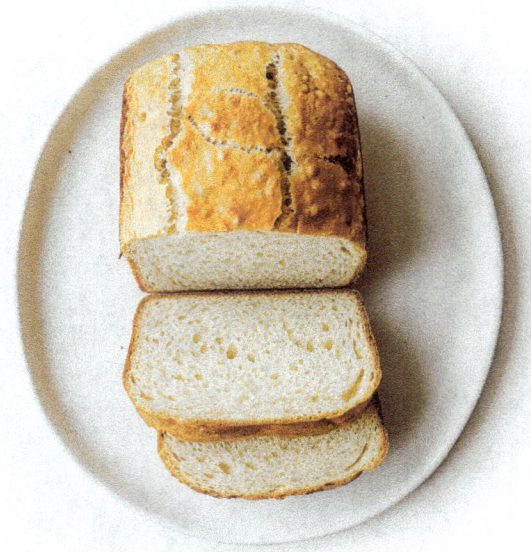

GLUTEN-FREE FLOUR BLEND

SERVES 4 cups

PREP 10 min

COOK n/a

READY IN 10 min

INGREDIENTS

2 cups white rice flour

1 cup tapioca flour

1 cup potato starch

2 teaspoons xanthan gum
(optional, if desired for
elasticity in baking)

DIRECTIONS

1. In a large mixing bowl, whisk together the white rice flour, tapioca flour, potato starch, and optional xanthan gum until well combined. Ensure that all ingredients are evenly distributed to create a uniform blend.

2. Transfer the flour blend to an airtight container. Seal the container tightly to prevent moisture from affecting the flour.

3. Before each use, shake the container well to redistribute the flours, as they may settle during storage.

4. Store the gluten-free flour blend in a cool, dry place away from direct sunlight. Properly stored, the blend should remain fresh for several months.

NOTE

- This blend can be used as a one-to-one substitute for recipes that call for gluten-free all-purpose flour, making it a versatile option for your gluten-free baking needs.

PER SERVING (about 1 cup) Calories: 575; Total fat: 1g; Protein: 4g; Carbohydrates: 129g; Fiber: 5g

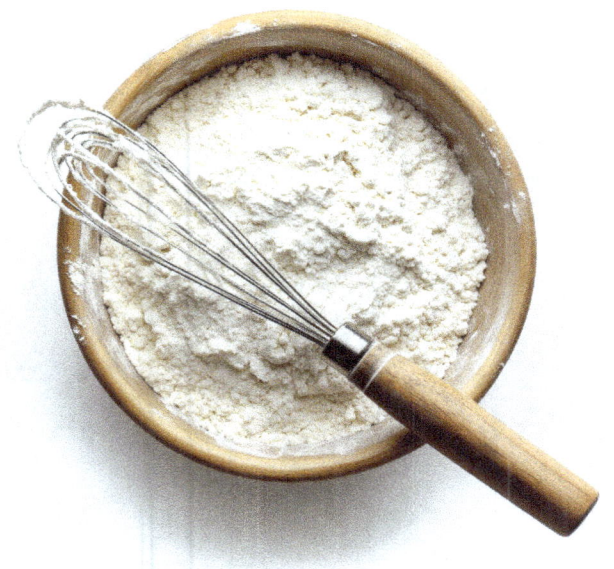

SPINACH WRAPS

SERVES 8 wraps

PREP 20 min

COOK 10 min

READY IN 30 min

INGREDIENTS

2 cups spinach leaves

2 cups oats (or oat flour)

3 cups water

1 teaspoon salt

DIRECTIONS

1. Boil water in a saucepan, add spinach, and cook until wilted. Blend into a smooth broth, strain, and reserve 2 cups.

2. In a bowl, mix oat flour and salt. Gradually stir in the hot spinach broth until well combined. Allow to cool.

3. Divide the dough into 8 pieces, roll into balls, and press each between parchment to form 8-10 inch discs.

4. Heat a non-stick skillet over medium-high. Cook tortillas for 30 seconds per side until puffed and golden.

5. Keep wraps warm under a cloth until ready to serve.

PER SERVING (1 wrap) Calories: 78; Total fat: 1g; Protein: 3g; Carbohydrates: 11g; Fiber: 2g

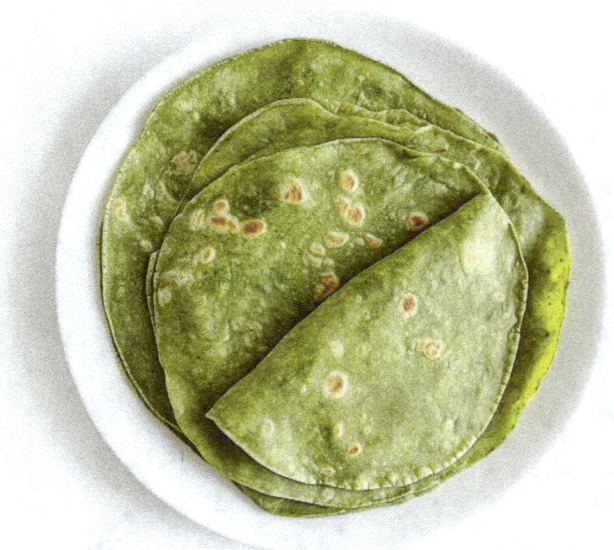

CASSAVA TORTILLAS

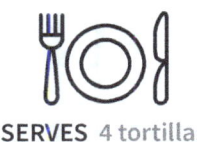

SERVES 4 tortillas

PREP 15 min

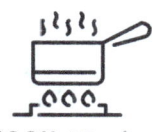

COOK 10 min

READY IN 25 min

INGREDIENTS

1 cup cassava flour

2 tablespoons olive oil

1 cup warm water

½ teaspoon salt

DIRECTIONS

1. In a mixing bowl, combine cassava flour with salt. Add olive oil and lukewarm water. Mix with your hands until a smooth dough forms.

2. Transfer the dough to a smooth surface and knead lightly until it becomes compact and no longer crumbles.

3. Divide the dough into 4 equal pieces and roll each into a ball.

4. Preheat a griddle over medium-high heat.

5. Prepare a tortilla press with two pieces of parchment paper. Place one dough ball between the parchment layers and press into a tortilla.

6. Carefully peel off the top parchment, flip the tortilla into your hand, and gently remove the second piece of parchment.

7. Immediately cook the tortilla on the preheated griddle. Allow it to cook until bubbles form, then flip it over and cook until browned on the other side. Avoid flipping the tortilla before bubbles form to prevent breaking.

8. Repeat the process with the remaining dough balls.

9. Serve the tortillas immediately, or keep them covered with a cloth. If needed, reheat in the microwave.

PER SERVING (1 tortilla) Calories: 164; Total fat: 6g; Protein: 2g; Carbohydrates: 24g; Fiber: 2g

CHICKEN BROTH

 **SERVES** 8 cups    **PREP** 10 min    **COOK** 2 hours    **READY IN** 2 h 10 min

INGREDIENTS

1 to 2 pounds chicken bones or parts (wings and necks are ideal)

2 medium carrots, coarsely chopped

2 celery stalks, coarsely chopped

1 bay leaves

2 sprigs fresh thyme (or ½ teaspoon dried thyme)

4 fresh parsley stems

8 cups water

¼ teaspoon asafoetida (optional)

½ teaspoon salt (optional)

PER SERVING (about 1 cup)
Calories: 12; Total fat: 0g; Protein: 0g;
Carbohydrates: 3g; Fiber: 0g

DIRECTIONS

1. In a large soup pot, combine chicken bones or parts, carrots, celery, bay leaves, parsley stems, and thyme.

2. Cover with water and bring to a boil over medium-high heat.

3. Reduce heat to medium-low and simmer, uncovered, for 2 hours to allow flavors and nutrients to be extracted.

4. Optional Slow Cooker Method: Alternatively, place all ingredients in a slow cooker and set to low for 24 hours.

5. Strain the broth through a fine sieve to remove solids.

6. Refrigerate overnight and skim off any fat that forms on the surface.

7. Store the broth in airtight containers in the refrigerator for up to 5 days or freeze for up to 6 months.

NOTE

- For a seafood version, replace chicken bones with fish bones to make a light fish stock, ideal for enhancing seafood dishes.

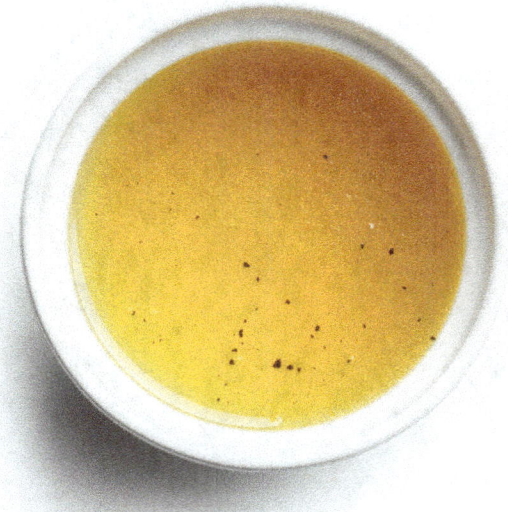

VEGETABLE BROTH

SERVES 8 cups

PREP 15 min

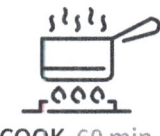

COOK 60 min

READY IN 1 h 15 min

INGREDIENTS

2 medium carrots, peeled and chopped

2 celery stalks, chopped

1 leek (white part only), rinsed and chopped

1 fennel bulb, chopped (optional, see notes)

2 bay leaves

3 sprigs fresh parsley

3 sprigs fresh thyme or 1 teaspoon dried thyme

8 cups water

½ teaspoon salt (optional)

DIRECTIONS

1. In a large pot, combine carrots, celery, leek, optional fennel, bay leaves, parsley, thyme, water, and salt (if using).

2. Bring to a boil over high heat, then reduce to a simmer, cover, and cook for 1 hour to allow flavors to meld.

3. Remove from heat and strain the broth using a fine-mesh sieve, discarding solids.

4. Let broth cool for about 30 minutes before transferring to glass containers for storage.

5. Refrigerate for up to one week or freeze for extended storage.

NOTE

- Omitting fennel won't compromise the overall flavor. Substitute with a pinch of fennel seeds for a similar effect if desired.

PER SERVING (about 1 cup) Calories: 8; Total fat: 0g; Protein: 0g; Carbohydrates: 2g; Fiber: 0g

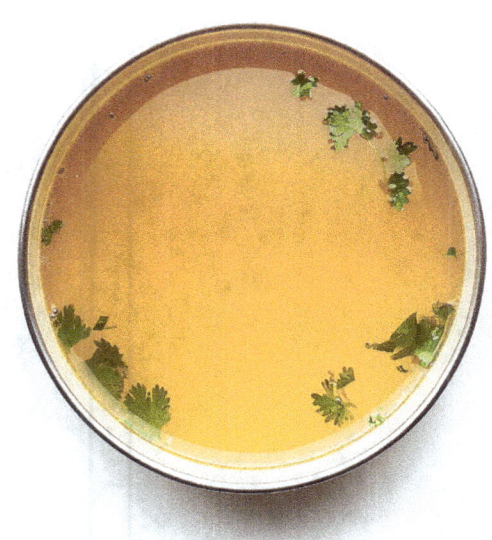

CREAMY HERB DRESSING

SERVES 2

PREP 5 min

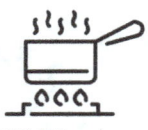
COOK n/a

READY IN 5 min

INGREDIENTS

½ cup non-dairy plain yogurt (see note for a healing phase substitute)

1 teaspoon grated lemon zest

1 tablespoon fresh parsley, chopped

1 tablespoon fresh thyme, chopped

1 teaspoon fresh rosemary, chopped

¼ teaspoon salt

DIRECTIONS

1. In a small bowl, combine all the ingredients. Mix well until everything is thoroughly blended.

NOTE

- For a healing phase alternative, substitute the non-dairy yogurt with ½ cup silken tofu and 2 tablespoons plant-based milk. Blend these ingredients in a food processor or blender until smooth, then add the herbs, zest, and salt, blending again to combine. Adjust the consistency with additional milk if necessary.

PER SERVING (about ¼ cup) Calories: 55; Total fat: 1g; Protein: 1g; Carbohydrates: 10g; Fiber: 1g

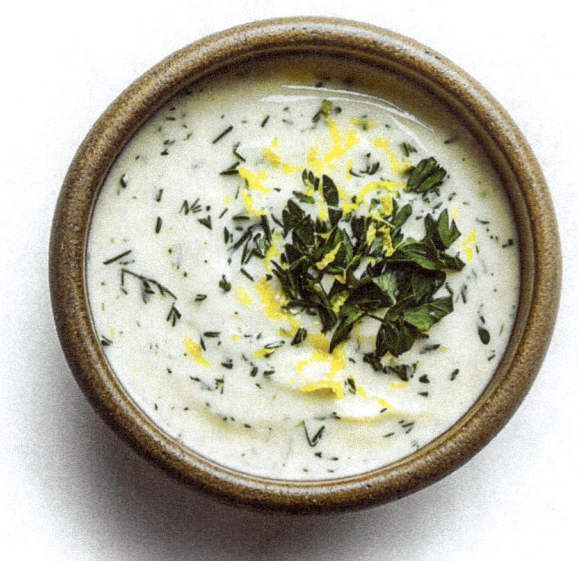

TOMATO-FREE PASTA SAUCE

 SERVES 4

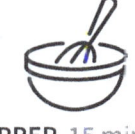 PREP 15 min

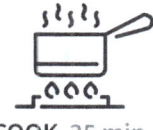 COOK 35 min

 READY IN 50 min

INGREDIENTS

1 cup carrots, diced (about 2 medium carrots)

1 cup butternut squash, cubed

1 cup celery, diced

1 medium beet, finely cubed

2 cups water

1 ½ tablespoons olive oil

1 teaspoon each of dried or fresh thyme, basil, oregano, and rosemary (increase to 1 tablespoon if fresh)

1 tablespoon grated lemon zest

1 teaspoon maple syrup or honey

¼ teaspoon asafoetida (optional)

1 teaspoon salt, more to taste

DIRECTIONS

1. Heat olive oil in a large stockpot over medium heat. Add the carrots, celery, and squash. Sauté for 4-5 minutes, stirring often. Add a splash of water if the vegetables begin to stick.

2. Add the beets, salt, and dried herbs (or fresh, if using). Continue to sauté for another 1-2 minutes.

3. Pour in the water, lemon zest, and maple syrup or honey. Bring the mixture to a low boil, then reduce the heat and cover.

4. Simmer on low for about 30 minutes, or until the carrots, beets, and squash are tender.

5. Remove from heat and let cool slightly. Using an immersion blender, blend the ingredients directly in the pot until smooth. Alternatively, carefully transfer the mixture to a blender and puree.

6. Taste and adjust the seasoning with additional salt as needed.

PER SERVING (about ½ cup) Calories: 106; Total fat: 5g; Protein: 1g; Carbohydrates: 11g; Fiber: 3g

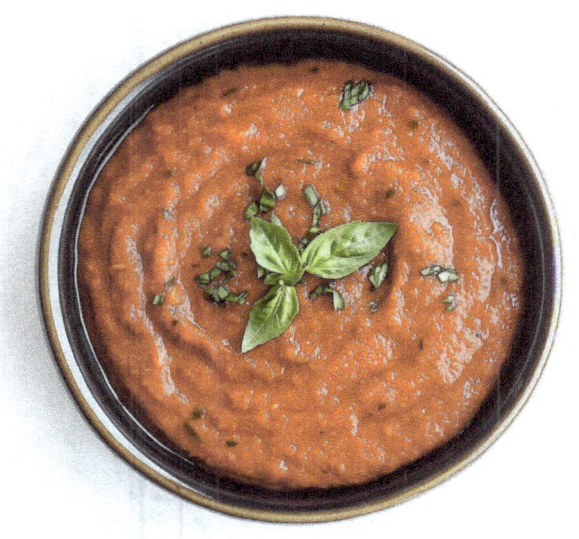

AVOCADO SAUCE

SERVES 4

PREP 5 min

COOK n/a

READY IN 5 min

INGREDIENTS

1 ripe avocado

¼ cup almond milk (or plain dairy-free yogurt for maintenance phase)

2 tablespoons fresh cilantro, chopped

Zest of 1 lime

¼ teaspoon salt (or to taste)

DIRECTIONS

1. Cut the avocado in half, remove the pit, and scoop out the flesh into a food processor.

2. Add the almond milk (or dairy-free yogurt), cilantro, lime zest, and salt to the food processor. Blend until smooth and creamy.

3. Taste the sauce and adjust seasoning if necessary, adding more salt or almond milk for consistency if desired.

4. Use this sauce as a topping for your tacos or a dip for other dishes.

NOTE

- You can adjust the thickness by adding more almond milk for a thinner sauce or less for a thicker consistency.

PER SERVING (about ¼ cup) Calories: 80; Total fat: 37g; Protein: 1g; Carbohydrates: 4g; Fiber: 3g

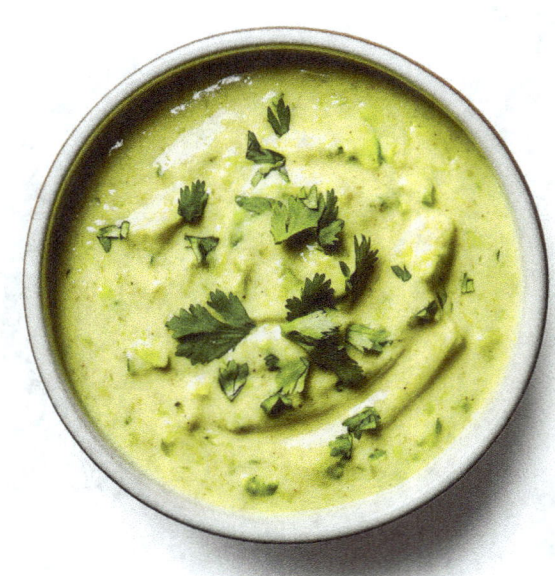

TZATZIKI SAUCE

SERVES 8

PREP 10 min

COOK n/a

READY IN 12 min

INGREDIENTS

½ cup raw unsalted cashews, soaked overnight

½ cup English cucumber, grated

⅓ cup water

1 tablespoon grated lemon zest

1 tablespoon fresh dill, chopped

½ teaspoon salt

DIRECTIONS

1. Rinse and drain the soaked cashews.

2. In a blender, combine the cashews, water, lemon zest, and salt. Blend on high speed until the mixture is completely smooth and creamy, about 1-2 minutes.

3. Add the grated cucumber and dill to the blender Pulse briefly, just until the cucumber is mixed through but still retains some texture and the dill is evenly distributed.

4. Transfer the sauce to an airtight container and refrigerate. Best if used on the same day.

NOTE

- Traditional tzatziki is made with dairy yogurt, which can be problematic for some stomachs. For a tangier flavor, substitute the cashews with ½ cup dairy-free yogurt if preferred.

PER SERVING (about 2 tablespoons) Calories: 45; Total fat: 3g; Protein: 1g; Carbohydrates: 2g; Fiber: 0g

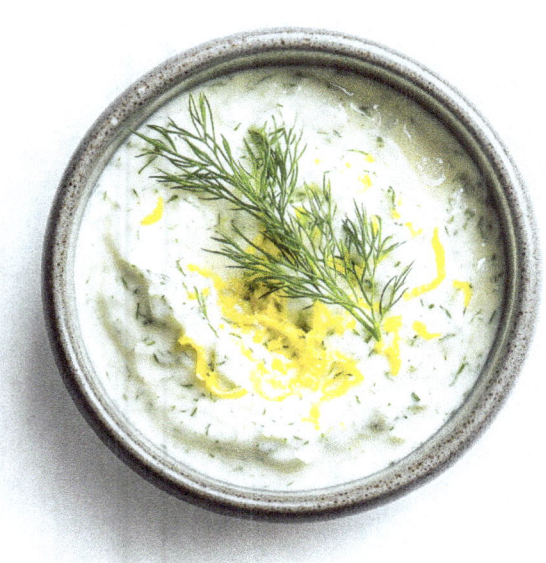

PAPAYA DRESSING

SERVES 6 **PREP** 10 min **COOK** n/a **READY IN** 12 min

INGREDIENTS

½ medium papaya, seeded, peeled, and cut into chunks

1½ tablespoons olive oil

1 teaspoon grated lemon zest

1 tablespoon fresh thyme, chopped

1 teaspoon maple syrup or honey

¼ cup water

½ teaspoon salt

DIRECTIONS

1. In a blender or food processor, add the papaya, olive oil, lemon zest, thyme, maple syrup (or honey), and salt.

2. Blend until the mixture is completely smooth. If the mixture is too thick, gradually add water to reach your desired consistency.

3. Taste and adjust seasoning if necessary.

PER SERVING (about 2 tablespoons)
Calories: 44; Total fat: 3g; Protein: 0g;
Carbohydrates: 3g; Fiber: 0g

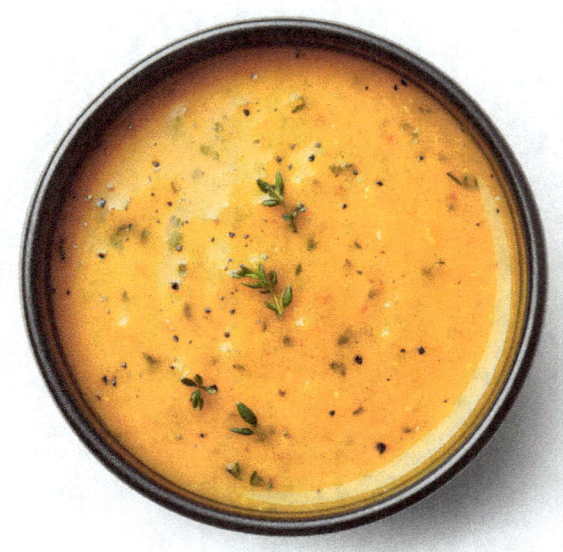

BUTTERNUT SQUASH PASTA SAUCE

SERVES 4

PREP 15 min

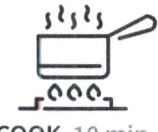
COOK 10 min

READY IN 25 min

INGREDIENTS

½ cup butternut squash, peeled and diced

1 medium carrot, peeled and chopped

2 tablespoons canned coconut milk

1 tablespoon nutritional yeast

½ teaspoon dried or fresh dill

A pinch of asafoetida (optional)

A small dash of liquid aminos or coconut aminos (optional, adjust to taste)

DIRECTIONS

1. Bring a small pot of water to a boil. Add the chopped carrot and butternut squash. Boil until they are soft and tender, about 10-12 minutes.

2. Drain the vegetables and transfer them to a blender or food processor. Add the coconut milk, nutritional yeast, dill, asafoetida, and a splash of liquid aminos.

3. Blend until the mixture is smooth and creamy. Add water to adjust the consistency if necessary.

4. Transfer the sauce to a saucepan and simmer over low heat for 2-3 minutes to meld the flavors. Taste and adjust the seasoning with salt or additional aminos if needed.

5. Serve over your favorite cooked pasta.

PER SERVING (about ¼ cup) Calories: 34; Total fat: 1g; Protein: 1g; Carbohydrates: 3g; Fiber: 1g

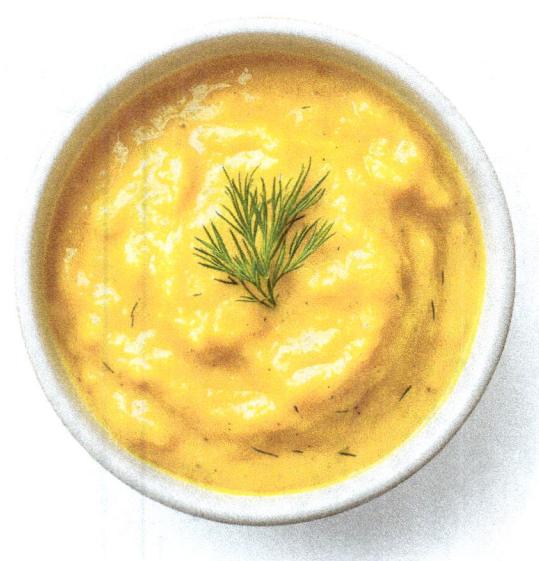

CREAMY CHEESE SAUCE

SERVES 6

PREP 15 min

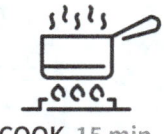

COOK 15 min

READY IN 30 min

INGREDIENTS

¾ cup potatoes, peeled and cubed

¾ cup sweet potatoes, peeled and cubed

¼ cup raw cashews (optional soaking, see note)

2 tablespoons olive oil

¼ cup water

1 tablespoon grated lemon zest

2 tablespoons nutritional yeast

¼ teaspoon asafoetida (optional, for depth)

½ teaspoon salt, or to taste

DIRECTIONS

1. In a pot, add the cubed potatoes and sweet potatoes, covering them with cold water. Sprinkle in a pinch of salt and bring to a boil. Once boiling, reduce to a simmer and cook until the vegetables are tender, typically 8-12 minutes.

2. Once the potatoes are soft, drain them and place them in a blender. Add the soaked cashews (if using), olive oil, water, lemon zest, nutritional yeast, asafoetida, and salt.

3. Blend on high until the mixture becomes completely smooth and creamy. You may need to pause and scrape down the sides to ensure everything mixes evenly.

4. The cheese sauce is now ready to serve! It's excellent as a dip or drizzled over dishes like pasta or steamed vegetables.

NOTE

- For those with standard blenders, soaking the cashews in warm water for 2 hours beforehand will help achieve a smoother blend. Simply drain them and proceed with the recipe. If you have a high-powered blender, you can skip this step.

PER SERVING (about ¼ cup) Calories: 127; Total fat: 7g; Protein: 3g; Carbohydrates: 11g; Fiber: 2g

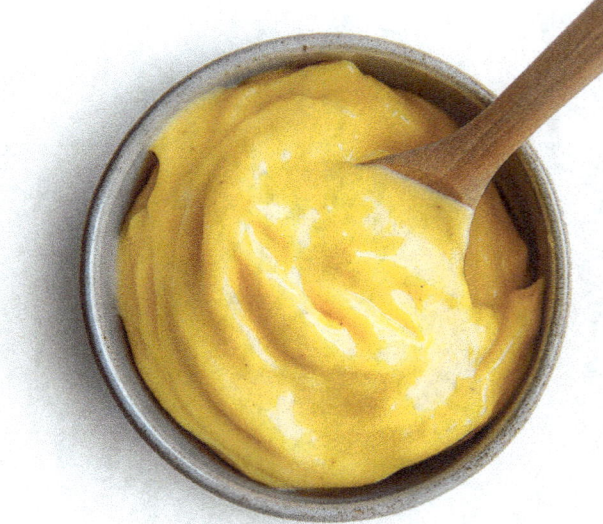

VEGAN PARMESAN CHEESE

SERVES 12

PREP 10 min

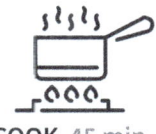
COOK 45 min

READY IN 55 min

INGREDIENTS

1 cup potato starch

¼ cup refined coconut oil, melted

½ cup unsweetened almond milk (or any plant-based milk)

⅓ cup nutritional yeast

1 tablespoon white miso paste

1 tablespoon freshly grated lemon zest

1 ½ teaspoons salt

DIRECTIONS

1. Combine all ingredients in a high-speed blender. Blend until the texture is completely smooth, scraping down the sides of the blender as necessary to ensure an even mix.

2. Lightly grease a heat-safe dish that holds at least 2 cups (500 ml) and fits inside a steamer basket. Transfer the Parmesan mixture into the dish and cover tightly with aluminum foil.

3. Prepare a steamer setup by filling a large pot with several inches of water and bringing it to a boil. Place the covered dish inside the steamer basket, cover the pot with a lid, and let steam for 35 to 45 minutes. The cheese should be firm and springy to the touch, and slightly darker in color.

4. After steaming, remove the dish and allow it to cool slightly. If there's any condensation on the surface, pat it dry with a paper towel.

5. Refrigerate the cheese overnight to set completely. If needed, run a knife along the edges of the dish to loosen the Parmesan before unmolding.

6. Shape the Parmesan into a rustic wedge by scoring with a knife and breaking it along the scored lines for a natural look.

7. Enjoy your vegan Parmesan by grating or slicing it over dishes. It can be refrigerated for up to two weeks or frozen for three months in an airtight container.

PER SERVING (about 2 tablespoons) Calories: 115; Total fat: 5g; Protein: 1g; Carbohydrates: 14g; Fiber: 1g

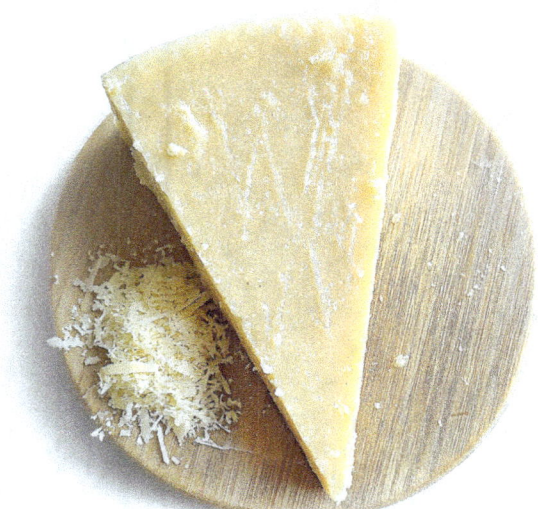

TOFU CREAM CHEESE

 SERVES 4-6

 PREP 10 min

 COOK n/a

 READY IN 10 min

INGREDIENTS

7 oz (200 g) extra-firm tofu

2 tablespoons nutritional yeast

1 teaspoon finely grated lemon zest

¼ teaspoon salt

1 tablespoon finely chopped fresh dill (or frozen, thawed)

2–4 tablespoons unsweetened non-dairy milk

DIRECTIONS

1. Crumble the tofu and press out excess moisture if needed. If your tofu isn't pre-pressed, wrap it in a clean kitchen towel and place a heavy object on top for about 10 minutes.

2. Transfer the tofu to a blender or food processor. Add the nutritional yeast, lemon zest, salt, dill, and 2 tablespoons of non-dairy milk. Blend until smooth and creamy, pausing to scrape down the sides as necessary.

3. Adjust consistency by adding more non-dairy milk, one tablespoon at a time. Taste and tweak the flavor—more nutritional yeast for cheesiness, a bit of extra zest for brightness, or additional dill for a bolder herb flavor.

4. Transfer to a container and refrigerate for at least 2 hours to allow the texture to firm up and the flavors to develop.

5. Store in an airtight container in the refrigerator for up to 1 week. Stir before each use if needed.

NOTE

- For a firmer, richer spread, you can blend in 2 tablespoons of coconut oil with the other ingredients. This helps the mixture set more firmly once chilled. However, keep in mind it will increase the fat content.

PER SERVING (about 2 tablespoons)
Calories: 32; Total fat: 1.7g; Protein: 3.9g; Carbohydrates: 0.3g; Fiber: 0g

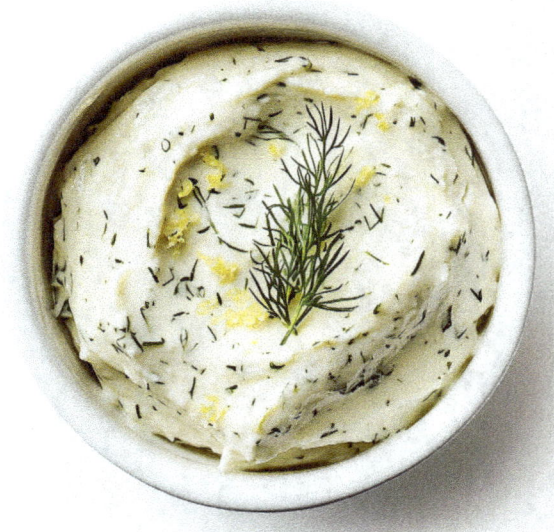

CASHEW MAYONNAISE

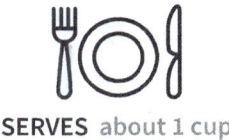 **SERVES** about 1 cup

 **PREP** 5 min

 **COOK** n/a

 **READY IN** 10 min

INGREDIENTS

1 cup raw cashews (soaked for 2–4 hours, then drained)

1 cup water

½ teaspoon salt

½ teaspoon honey (or maple syrup for vegan option)

1 teaspoon chia seeds

Optional: finely grated zest of ½ lemon, for added brightness

DIRECTIONS

1. Place all ingredients in a high-speed blender or food processor. Blend on high until smooth and velvety, scraping down the sides as needed. Adjust seasoning to taste—add more salt, lemon zest, or sweetener if desired.

2. Refrigerate for 30 minutes before serving to allow the chia seeds to thicken the mayo and develop flavor.

3. Store in an airtight container in the refrigerator for up to 5–6 days. Stir before each use, as slight separation may occur.

PER SERVING (about 2 tablespoons) Calories: 90; Total fat: 6.4g; Protein: 2.9g; Carbohydrates: 5.6g; Fiber: 0.8g

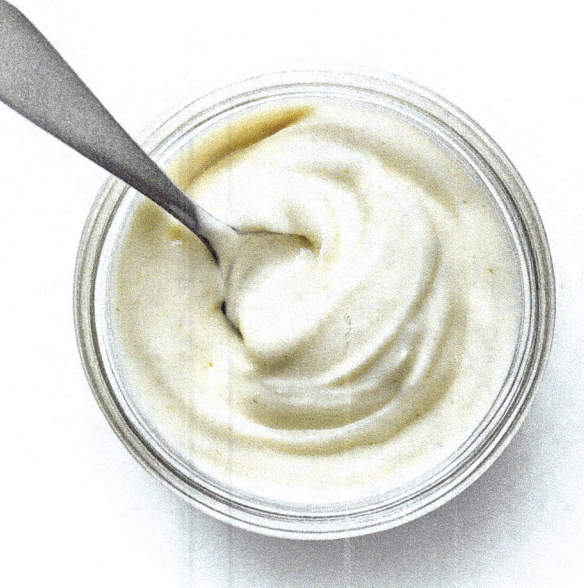

DATE SYRUP

SERVES 1½ to 2 cups

PREP 15 min

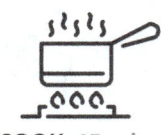

COOK 45 min

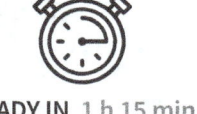

READY IN 1 h 15 min

INGREDIENTS

1 pound Medjool dates, pitted (about 2 ½ to 3 cups packed)

3 cups boiling water (plus more as needed)

DIRECTIONS

1. Place the dates in a saucepan and pour in the boiling water. Let soak for 15 minutes.

2. Once softened, bring the mixture to a boil, then reduce to a simmer. Cook for 15 minutes, mashing the dates occasionally and stirring to prevent sticking. The mixture should resemble loose applesauce.

3. Let cool slightly, then transfer to a nut milk bag or cheesecloth over a bowl. Squeeze out all the liquid, leaving behind the pulp.

4. Return the strained liquid to the pot and simmer on low for 20–30 minutes, stirring often, until it thickens into a syrup. If it gets too thick, add a splash of water to loosen.

5. Cool completely and store in a sealed jar in the fridge for up to 2 weeks.

PER SERVING (about 1 tablespoon)
Calories: 44; Total fat: 0g; Protein: 0.3g;
Carbohydrates: 10.8g; Fiber: 1g

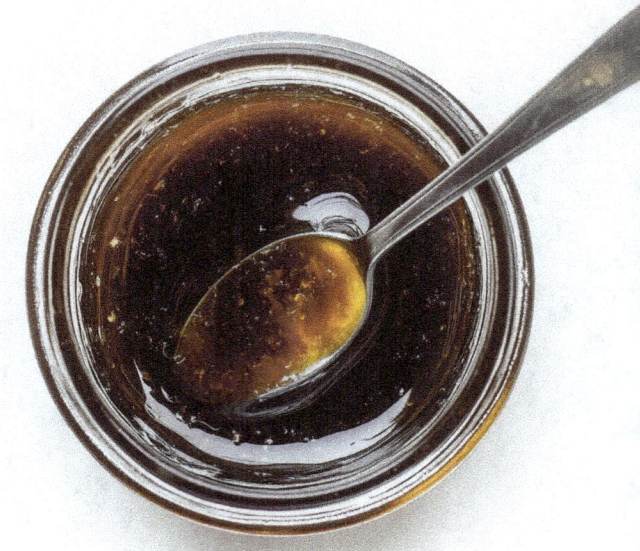

RANCH DRESSING

SERVES 4

PREP 5 min

COOK n/a

READY IN 5 min

INGREDIENTS

¼ cup unsweetened non-dairy milk

¼ cup plain non-dairy yogurt (almond, coconut, or cashew-based)

2 tablespoons finely chopped fresh dill

Zest of 1 lemon

½ teaspoon salt

DIRECTIONS

1. Add all ingredients to a blender or food processor. Blend until smooth and creamy, scraping down the sides as needed. Taste and adjust salt or lemon zest to your liking.

2. Use immediately or chill for 30 minutes to enhance the flavor. Store leftovers in an airtight container in the refrigerator for up to 3 days.

PER SERVING (about 2 tablespoons) Calories: 16; Total fat: 0.5g; Protein: 0.2g; Carbohydrates: 2.7g; Fiber: 0.3g

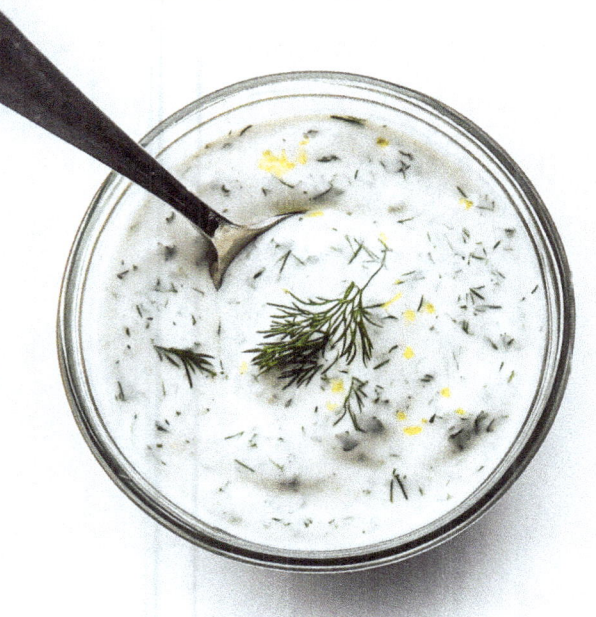

MEASUREMENTS AND CONVERSIONS

VOLUMEN EQUIVALENTS (LIQUID)		
US STANDARDS	**US STANDARDS (OUNCES)**	**METRIC (APPROX.)**
2 tablespoons	1 fl. oz.	30 mL
¼ cup	2 fl. oz.	60 mL
½ cup	4 fl. oz.	120 mL
1 cup	8 fl. oz.	240 mL
1 ½ cups	12 fl. oz.	355 mL
2 cups or 1 pint	16 fl. oz.	475 mL
4 cups or 1 quart	32 fl. oz.	1 L
1 gallon	128 fl. oz.	4 L

VOLUMEN EQUIVALENTS (DRY)	
US STANDARDS	**METRIC (APPROX.)**
⅛ teaspoon	0.5 mL
¼ teaspoon	1 mL
½ teaspoon	2 mL
¾ teaspoon	4 mL
1 teaspoon	5 mL
1 tablespoon	15 mL
¼ cup	59 mL

⅓ cup	79 mL
½ cup	118 mL
⅔ cup	156 mL
¾ cup	177 mL
1 cup	235 mL
2 cups or 1 pint	475 mL
3 cups	700 mL
4 cups or 1 quart	1 L

WEIGHT EQUIVALENTS

US STANDARD	METRIC (APPROX.)
½ ounce	15 g
1 ounce	30 g
2 ounces	60 g
4 ounces	115 g
8 ounces	225 g
12 ounces	340 g
16 ounces or 1 pound	455 g

OVEN TEMPERATURES

FAHRENHEIT (F)	CELSIUS (C) (APPROX.)
250°F	120°C
300°F	150°C
325°F	165°C
350°F	180°C
375°F	190°C
400°F	200°C
425°F	220°C
450°F	230°C

THE pH LEVEL FOOD LISTS

FRUITS	pH
Acai Berries	4.4 to 4.6
Apples (Gala, Red Delicious)	4.3 to 4.8
Apricots	3.5 to 4.8
Avocado	6.3 to 6.6
Banana, yellow	5.0 to 5.7
Blackberries	3.2 to 3.6
Blackcurrants	2.8 to 3.6
Blueberries	3.5 to 4.3
Boysenberries	3.2 to 3.6
Cantaloupe	6.1 to 6.6
Cherries	3.2 to 4.5
Clementines	3.2 to 4.0
Cranberries	2.3 to 2.5
Dates (Medjool, Deglet Noor)	5.4 to 5.7
Dragon fruit	5.0 to 5.4
Elderberries	3.5 to 4.5
Fig, Calimyrna	5.0 to 5.9
Grapefruit	2.9 to 3.3
Grapes	3.3 to 4.2
Gooseberries	2.8 to 3.3

Guava	2.9 to 4.9
Green apple (Granny Smith)	3.3 to 4.0
Jackfruit	4.6 to 5.2
Jujube	4.6 to 5.2
Kiwi	3.1 to 4.0
Kumquat	3.6 to 4.8
Lemon	2.2 to 2.4
Lemon zest	5.0 to 5.7
Lime	2.0 to 2.8
Lime zest	5.0 to 5.6
Lychee	4.4 to 5.6
Mangoes	3.4 to 4.8
Melons	5.4 to 6.6
Mulberries	3.4 to 4.4
Nectarines	3.9 to 4.1
Olives, black	5.4 to 6.5
Olives, green (fermented)	3.6 to 4.2
Orange zest	5.5 to 6.0
Oranges	3.1 to 4.1
Papaya	5.2 to 5.7
Peaches	3.3 to 4.2
Pear (Bartlett, Forelle)	4.0 to 4.6
Pear, Asian	5.3 to 5.7
Pear, Bosc	5.1 to 5.3
Passion fruit	2.8 to 3.2
Pineapple	3.2 to 4.0
Pineberries	3.0 to 4.0
Plantain	4.9 to 5.5
Plums	2.8 to 4.4
Pomegranates	2.9 to 3.2
Prunes	3.6 to 3.9
Pumpkin	5.0 to 5.5

Quince	3.3 to 4.4
Raisins	3.5 to 4.5
Raspberries	3.2 to 3.7
Soursop	3.8 to 4.3
Starfruit (Carambola)	2.5 to 3.7
Strawberries	3.0 to 3.8
Tangerines	3.2 to 4.4
Watermelon	5.2 to 5.8

VEGETABLES AND HERBS	pH
Acorn squash	5.0 to 6.0
Arugula	5.8 to 6.0
Artichoke	5.5 to 6.0
Asparagus	6.0 to 6.7
Bamboo shoots	5.1 to 6.2
Basil	5.5 to 6.2
Beet	5.3 to 6.6
Bell peppers	4.6 to 5.4
Bok Choy	6.0 to 6.7
Broccoli	6.3 to 6.5
Brussels sprouts	6.0 to 6.3
Butternut squash	5.5 to 5.9
Cabbage	5.4 to 6.2
Carrot	5.8 to 6.4
Cauliflower	5.5 to 6.8
Celeriac	5.8 to 6.5
Celery	5.7 to 6.0
Chard	6.1 to 6.7
Chayote	6.0 to 6.3
Chives	5.2 to 6.1
Collard greens	6.0 to 6.8

Cucumber	5.1 to 5.7
Eggplant	4.5 to 5.3
Endive	5.7 to 6.0
Fennel	5.8 to 6.0
Garlic	5.8 to 6.5
Ginger	5.6 to 6.2
Hearts of palm	5.0 to 6.7
Horseradish	5.5 to 6.8
Jerusalem artichoke	5.5 to 6.2
Jicama	5.5 to 6.5
Kale	6.0 to 6.2
Kohlrabi	5.5 to 5.8
Leek	5.5 to 6.2
Lemongrass	5.4 to 5.6
Lettuce	5.8 to 6.3
Mushroom	6.0 to 6.7
Mustard greens	5.5 to 6.3
Okra	5.5 to 6.4
Onion	5.3 to 5.8
Parsley	5.7 to 6.0
Parsnip	5.3 to 5.8
Peppers (hot varieties)	4.6 to 5.4
Potato	5.4 to 6.1
Radishes	5.5 to 6.0
Rhubarb	3.1 to 3.4
Rutabaga	5.2 to 5.7
Scallions	5.3 to 5.8
Sorrel	3.5 to 4.5
Spinach	5.5 to 6.8
Summer squash	5.5 to 6.2
Sweet potato	5.3 to 5.6

Taro	5.0 to 5.5
Tomato	4.2 to 4.9
Turnip	5.2 to 5.9
Watercress	6.5 to 7.0
Zucchini	5.7 to 6.1

GRAINS AND LEGUMES	pH
Amaranth	6.5 to 7.0
Barley	5.1 to 5.3
Beans	5.4 to 6.5
Brown rice	6.2 to 6.7
Buckwheat	6.0 to 6.5
Chickpea	6.4 to 6.8
Corn	5.9 to 7.3
Edamame	6.0 to 6.5
Farro	6.0 to 6.5
Green beans	5.7 to 6.2
Kamut	6.0 to 6.5
Lentils	6.3 to 6.8
Millet	6.2 to 6.5
Oatmeal (cooked)	6.2 to 6.6
Oats	5.3 to 5.9
Peas	5.8 to 6.8
Quinoa	6.2 to 6.8
Rye	5.8 to 6.2
Sorghum	5.5 to 6.5
Soy	6.0 to 6.6
Spelt	5.4 to 6.1
Teff	5.9 to 6.5
White rice	6.0 to 6.7
Whole wheat	5.5 to 6.5
Wild rice	6.0 to 6.4

NUTS AND SEEDS	pH
Almonds	6.0 to 6.9
Brazil nuts	6.4 to 6.8
Cashews	5.7 to 6.2
Chestnuts	5.1 to 6.0
Chia seeds	6.5 to 7.2
Coconut	6.5 to 7.2
Flaxseed	6.4 to 7.0
Hazelnuts	5.3 to 6.0
Hemp seeds	6.0 to 6.5
Macadamia nuts	5.2 to 6.2
Pecans (roasted)	5.6 to 6.4
Pine nuts	6.5 to 7.0
Pistachios	6.0 to 6.4
Pumpkin seeds	5.5 to 6.5
Sesame seeds	6.6 to 7.1
Sunflower seeds	6.0 to 6.5
Walnuts, raw	5.8 to 6.4
Peanuts	6.3 to 6.8

MEAT, POULTRY, FISH, AND SEAFOOD	pH
Anchovies	6.3 to 6.8
Beef (ground)	5.3 to 5.7
Beef	5.8 to 7.0
Bison	5.4 to 5.8
Chicken	5.3 to 6.5
Clams	6.4 to 6.8
Cod	6.0 to 6.7
Crabmeat	6.5 to 7.0
Duck	5.7 to 6.4

Egg white	7.5 to 9.2
Egg yolk	6.3 to 6.7
Flounder (boiled)	6.1 to 6.9
Halibut	5.7 to 6.8
Lamb	5.4 to 6.7
Lobster (boiled)	7.0 to 7.4
Pork	5.4 to 5.8
Salmon (fresh)	6.1 to 6.3
Sardines (fresh)	6.5 to 7.1
Shrimp (boiled)	6.8 to 7.0
Tilapia (fresh)	6.0 to 6.2
Trout	6.3 to 6.8
Tuna (fresh)	5.2 to 6.1
Turkey	5.7 to 6.8
Veal	5.5 to 6.1
Venison	5.5 to 6.0

DAIRY PRODUCTS	pH
Blue Cheese	6.2 to 6.9
Butter (unsalted)	4.4 to 5.0
Buttermilk	4.4 to 4.8
Cheddar	5.1 to 5.9
Cream Cheese	4.5 to 4.9
Cottage Cheese	4.7 to 5.0
Gouda Cheese	5.0 to 5.6
Greek Yogurt	4.2 to 4.7
Heavy Cream	6.4 to 6.8
Ice Cream	5.8 to 6.6
Kefir	4.2 to 4.6
Milk	6.4 to 6.8
Mozzarella	5.1 to 5.4

Parmesan	5.2 to 5.9
Ricotta Cheese	5.1 to 5.4
Sour Cream	4.4 to 4.8
Whey	5.6 to 6.6
Yogurt	4.0 to 4.5

OTHER	pH
Agave nectar	4.2 to 4.8
Almond butter	6.0 to 6.5
Almond milk (homemade)	6.5 to 7.5
Cider	2.9 to 3.3
Coconut milk	6.1 to 7.0
Manuka honey	3.9 to 4.5
Maple syrup	5.6 to 7.5
Mayonnaise	3.8 to 4.5
Miso paste	4.9 to 5.3
Molasses	5.0 to 5.5
Mustard	3.5 to 4.6
Oat milk	6.0 to 6.5
Peanut butter	6.0 to 6.3
Raw honey	3.4 to 4.5
Rice milk	6.2 to 7.2
Sauerkraut	3.5 to 3.6
Soy milk	6.4 to 7.3
Soy sauce	4.4 to 5.4
Sunflower seed butter	6.0 to 6.5
Tahini	5.5 to 6.0
Tamari	4.9 to 5.2
Tofu	6.9 to 7.2
Tomato paste	3.5 to 4.7
Vinegar	2.4 to 3.4

Notes on the pH Values in Foods

When managing gastritis, understanding the pH levels in foods is crucial. As discussed in this book, foods with a pH below 5 can activate the pepsin enzyme, potentially aggravating the stomach lining. Recognizing which foods have high or low pH levels enables you to make dietary choices that aid your recovery process.

However, it's important to remember that pH levels in food can vary due to several factors—such as variety, ripeness, cultivation conditions, processing, and cooking. Therefore, although the foods on this list have been tested, the pH values listed here should be viewed only as approximations.

The only way to know the pH level of the foods you buy, whether at the supermarket or from a local farmer, is by measuring their pH with a food pH meter or similar equipments. This might mean you need to don your scientist's coat and start conducting tests. However, it might not be necessary to go through such lengths, as using the previous lists of foods and considering factors like variety, ripeness, and processing, you can make good dietary choices. For example, when purchasing fruits, ensure they are fully ripe as unripe fruits tend to be more acidic. Also, be aware that different varieties of the same food can have varying pH levels. For instance, a Granny Smith apple is typically more acidic compared to a Red Delicious.

Additionally, how food is processed can alter its pH. For instance, canned vegetables might have a different pH than fresh ones, which can also impact their effect on your stomach. By understanding these nuances, you can better manage your diet to minimize discomfort and promote healing during your recovery from gastritis.

REFERENCES

1. Teyssen S, González-Calero G, Schimiczek M, S. M. Maleic acid and succinic acid in fermented alcoholic beverages are the stimulants of gastric acid secretion. J. Clin. Invest. 103, 707–13 (1999).

2. Liszt KI, Ley JP, Lieder B, Behrens M, Stöger 2, Reiner A, Hochkogler CM, Köck E, Marchiori A, Hans J, Widder S, Krammer G, Sanger GJ, Somoza MM, Meyerhof W, S. V. Caffeine induces gastric acid secretion via bitter taste signaling in gastric parietal cells. Proc. Natl. Acad. Sci. 114, E6260–E6269 (2017).

3. Harris, J. B., Nigon, K., & Alonso, D. Adenosine-3',5'-monophosphate: intracellular mediator for methyl xanthine stimulation of gastric secretion. Gastroenterology, 57(4), 377–384. (1969).

4. He M, Sun J, Jiang ZQ, Y. Y. Effects of cow's milk beta-casein variants on symptoms of milk intolerance in Chinese adults: a multicentre, randomized controlled study. Nutr. J. 16, 72 (2017).

5. Philip, A., & White, N. D. Gluten, Inflammation, and Neurodegeneration. American journal of lifestyle medicine, 16(1), 32–35. https://doi.org/10.1177/15598276211049345 (2022).

ACKNOWLEDGMENTS

I'm truly thankful to so many people who have supported me through this journey.

First off, a huge thanks to my family. Your patience and understanding have given me the time and space I needed to create this book. Your constant support has been the foundation of my motivation.

A big shout-out to everyone at The Gastritis Healing Group. Your stories, challenges, and victories haven't just inspired this book, they've also created a sense of community that we all share. This book is as much yours as it is mine.

Thanks to my publishing team for your expert advice and steady support. Your excitement about this project has kept me going.

And to you, the reader, looking for comfort and healing: I'm so grateful for your trust. I hope this book helps you on your path to better health.

RECIPE INDEX

INDEX

ABOUT THE AUTHOR

L.G. CAPELLAN is a former chronic gastritis sufferer and the founder of TheGastritisBlog.com. In 2013, he was diagnosed with chronic gastritis and bile reflux, conditions he endured for years with little to no relief from conventional treatments. Frustrated and determined to find a solution, he took matters into his own hands, embarking on an intensive research journey to understand and heal his condition.

Over five years, he dedicated countless hours reading and scrutinizing medical texts, scientific studies, and trusted medical blogs and websites. His rigorous research and personal experiences granted him profound knowledge about gastritis, enabling him to develop a comprehensive healing program that successfully resolved his chronic stomach issues.

Today, he shares his wisdom and knowledge with others facing similar struggles. Through his supportive Facebook group, *The Gastritis Healing Group*, along with his informative blog and must-read book on gastritis, he offers guidance, support, and inspiration to individuals seeking to overcome their stomach issues and reclaim their health.

For more information or to connect with the author, see the contact details on the next page.

CONTACT AND FOLLOW

If you're looking to get in touch, share feedback, or have questions, the best way to contact the author is via email at contact@lgcapellan.com. You can also:

JOIN HIS COMMUNITY ON FACEBOOK:

The Gastritis Healing Group

FOLLOW HIM ON SOCIAL MEDIA:

Facebook - L.G. Capellan

Instagram - @lg_capellan

Twitter - @lg_capellan

EXPLORE MORE ON HIS BLOG AND WEBSITE:

TheGastritisBlog.com

LGCapellan.com

ALSO BY L.G. CAPELLAN

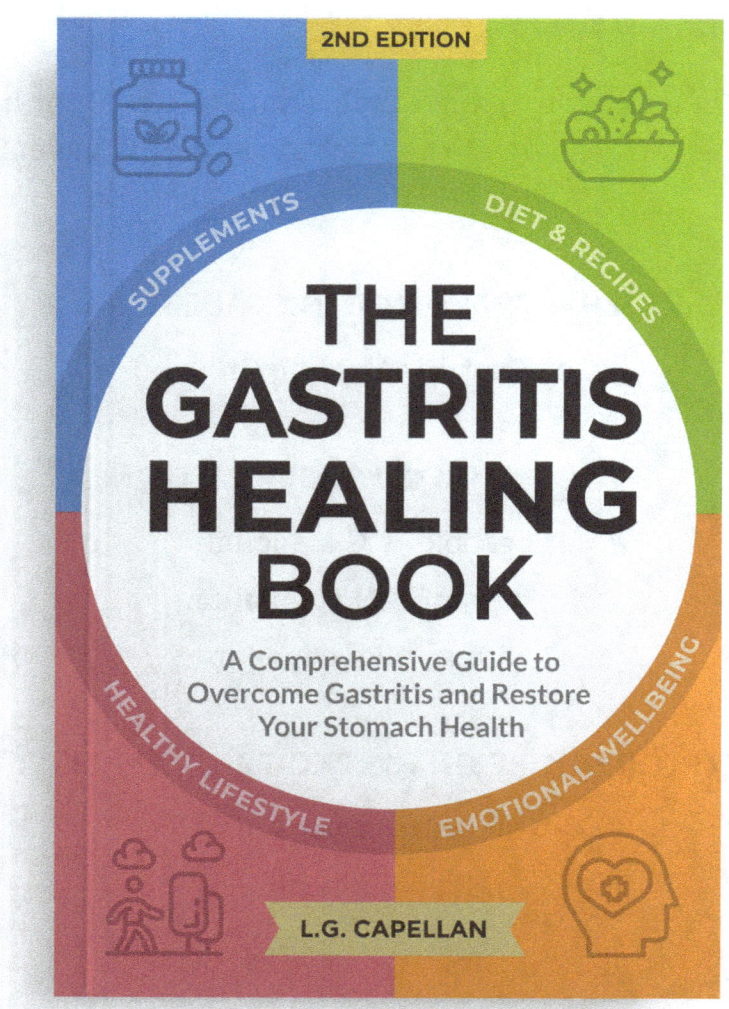

GET A FREE SAMPLE HERE:

LGCapellan.com/booksample